MW00824159

The Ultimate Mediterranean Cookbook

800 Easy and Healthy Mediterranean Recipes for Busy People to Make
Most Wanted Family Meals

By Tara B. Martinez

Copyright© 2021 By Tara B. Martinez

All Rights Reserved

The content contained within this book may not be reproduced, duplicated or transmitted without direct written permission from the author or the publisher.

Under no circumstances will any blame or legal responsibility be held against the publisher, or author, for any damages, reparation, or monetary loss due to the information contained within this book, either directly or indirectly.

Legal Notice:

This book is copyright protected. It is only for personal use. You cannot amend, distribute, sell, use, quote or paraphrase any part, or the content within this book, without the consent of the author or publisher.

Disclaimer Notice:

Please note the information contained within this document is for educational and entertainment purposes only. All effort has been executed to present accurate, up to date, reliable, complete information. No warranties of any kind are declared or implied. Readers acknowledge that the author is not engaged in the rendering of legal, financial, medical or professional advice. The content within this book has been derived from various sources. Please consult a licensed professional before attempting any techniques outlined in this book.

By reading this document, the reader agrees that under no circumstances is the author responsible for any losses, direct or indirect, that are incurred as a result of the use of the information contained within this document, including, but not limited to, errors, omissions, or inaccuracies.

Table of Content

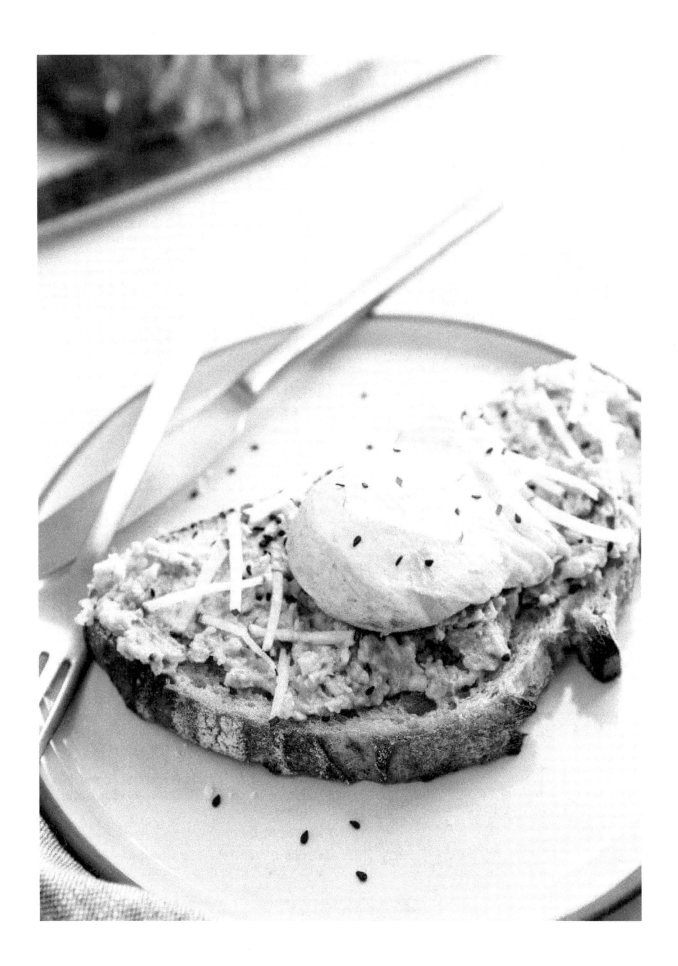

Chapter 1 Breakfasts

Veggie Stuffed Hash Browns

Prep time: 10 minutes | Cook time: 20 minutes | Serves 4

Ingredients:

Olive oil cooking spray
1 tablespoon plus 2 teaspoons olive oil, divided
4 ounces (113 g) baby bella mushrooms, diced
1 scallion, white parts and green parts, diced
1 garlic clove, minced
2 cups shredded potatoes
½ teaspoon salt
¼ teaspoon black pepper
1 Roma tomato, diced
½ cup shredded Mozzarella

Directions:

1. Preheat the air fryer to 380ºF (193ºC). Lightly coat the inside of a 6-inch cake pan with olive oil cooking spray.
2. In a small skillet, heat 2 teaspoons olive oil over medium heat. Add the mushrooms, scallion, and garlic, and cook for 4 to 5 minutes, or until they have softened and are beginning to show some color. Remove from heat.
3. Meanwhile, in a large bowl, combine the potatoes, salt, pepper, and the remaining tablespoon olive oil. Toss until all potatoes are well coated.
4. Pour half of the potatoes into the bottom of the cake pan. Top with the mushroom mixture, tomato, and Mozzarella. Spread the remaining potatoes over the top.
5. Bake in the air fryer for 12 to 15 minutes, or until the top is golden brown.
6. Remove from the air fryer and allow to cool for 5 minutes before slicing and serving.

Per Serving

calories: 164 | fat: 9g | protein: 6g
carbs: 16g | fiber: 3g | sodium: 403mg

Tomato, Herb, and Goat Cheese Frittata

Prep time: 15 minutes | Cook time: 25 minutes | Serves 2

Ingredients:

1 tablespoon olive oil
½ pint cherry or grape tomatoes
2 garlic cloves, minced
5 large eggs, beaten
3 tablespoons unsweetened almond milk
½ teaspoon salt
Pinch freshly ground
black pepper
2 tablespoons minced fresh oregano
2 tablespoons minced fresh basil
2 ounces (57 g) crumbled goat cheese (about ½ cup)

Directions:

1. Heat the oil in a nonstick skillet over medium heat. Add the tomatoes. As they start to cook, pierce some of them so they give off some of their juice. Reduce the heat to medium-low, cover the pan, and let the tomatoes soften.
2. When the tomatoes are mostly softened and broken down, remove the lid, add the garlic and continue to sauté.
3. In a medium bowl, combine the eggs, milk, salt, pepper, and herbs and whisk well to combine.
4. Turn the heat up to medium-high. Add the egg mixture to the tomatoes and garlic, then sprinkle the goat cheese over the eggs.
5. Cover the pan and let cook for about 7 minutes.
6. Uncover the pan and continue cooking for another 7 to 10 minutes, or until the eggs are set. Run a spatula around the edge of the pan to make sure they won't stick.
7. Let the frittata cool for about 5 minutes before serving. Cut it into wedges and serve.

Per Serving

calories: 417 | fat: 31g | protein: 26g
carbs: 12g | fiber: 3g | sodium: 867mg

Cheesy Mini Frittatas

Prep time: 10 minutes | Cook time: 25 minutes | Serves 6

Ingredients:

Nonstick cooking spray
1½ tablespoons extra-virgin olive oil
¼ cup chopped red potatoes (about 3 small)
¼ cup minced onions
¼ cup chopped red bell pepper
¼ cup asparagus, sliced lengthwise in half and chopped
4 large eggs
4 large egg whites
½ cup unsweetened almond milk
Salt and freshly ground black pepper, to taste
½ cup shredded low-moisture, part-skim Mozzarella cheese, divided

Directions:

1. Preheat the oven to 350ºF (180ºC). Using nonstick cooking spray, prepare a 12-count muffin pan.
2. In a medium sauté pan or skillet, heat the oil over medium heat and sauté the potatoes and onions for about 4 minutes, until the potatoes are fork-tender.
3. Add the bell pepper and asparagus and sauté for about 4 minutes, until just tender. Transfer the contents of a pan onto a paper-towel-lined plate to cool. In a bowl, whisk together the eggs, egg whites, and milk. Season with salt and pepper.
4. Once the vegetables are cooled to room temperature, add the vegetables and ¼ cup of Mozzarella cheese.
5. Using a spoon or ladle, evenly distribute the contents of the bowl into the prepared muffin pan, filling the cups about halfway.
6. Sprinkle the remaining ¼ cup of cheese over the top of the cups.
7. Bake for 20 to 25 minutes, or until eggs reach an internal temperature of 145ºF (63ºC) or the center is solid.
8. Allow the mini frittatas to rest for 5 to 10 minutes before removing from muffin pan and serving.

Per Serving (2 mini frittatas)

calories: 133 | fat: 9g | protein: 10g
carbs: 4g | fiber: 1g | sodium: 151mg

Avocado Toast with Poached Eggs

Prep time: 5 minutes | Cook time: 7 minutes | Serves 4

Ingredients:

Olive oil cooking spray
4 large eggs
Salt and black pepper, to taste
4 pieces whole grain bread
1 avocado
Red pepper flakes (optional)

Directions:

1. Preheat the air fryer to 320ºF (160ºC). Lightly coat the inside of four small oven-safe ramekins with olive oil cooking spray.
2. Crack one egg into each ramekin, and season with salt and black pepper.
3. Place the ramekins into the air fryer basket. Close and set the timer to 7 minutes.
4. While the eggs are cooking, toast the bread in a toaster.
5. Slice the avocado in half lengthwise, remove the pit, and scoop the flesh into a small bowl. Season with salt, black pepper, and red pepper flakes, if desired. Using a fork, smash the avocado lightly.
6. Spread a quarter of the smashed avocado evenly over each slice of toast.
7. Remove the eggs from the air fryer, and gently spoon one onto each slice of avocado toast before serving.

Per Serving

calories: 232 | fat: 14g | protein: 11g
carbs: 18g | fiber: 6g | sodium: 175mg

Prosciutto Breakfast Bruschetta

Prep time: 10 minutes | Cook time: 20 minutes | Serves 4

Ingredients:

¼ teaspoon kosher or sea salt
6 cups broccoli rabe, stemmed and chopped (about 1 bunch)
1 tablespoon extra-virgin olive oil
2 garlic cloves, minced (about 1 teaspoon)
1 ounce (28 g) prosciutto, cut or torn into ½-inch pieces
¼ teaspoon crushed red pepper
Nonstick cooking spray
3 large eggs
1 tablespoon unsweetened almond milk
¼ teaspoon freshly ground black pepper
4 teaspoons grated Parmesan or Pecorino Romano cheese
1 garlic clove, halved
8 (¾-inch-thick) slices baguette-style whole-grain bread or 4 slices larger Italian-style whole-grain bread

Directions:

1. Bring a large stockpot of water to a boil. Add the salt and broccoli rabe, and boil for 2 minutes. Drain in a colander.
2. In a large skillet over medium heat, heat the oil. Add the garlic, prosciutto, and crushed red pepper, and cook for 2 minutes, stirring often. Add the broccoli rabe and cook for an additional 3 minutes, stirring a few times. Transfer to a bowl and set aside.
3. Place the skillet back on the stove over low heat and coat with nonstick cooking spray.
4. In a small bowl, whisk together the eggs, milk, and pepper. Pour into the skillet. Stir and cook until the eggs are soft scrambled, 3 to 5 minutes. Add the broccoli rabe mixture back to the skillet along with the cheese. Stir and cook for about 1 minute, until heated through. Remove from the heat.
5. Toast the bread, then rub the cut sides of the garlic clove halves onto one side of each slice of the toast. (Save the garlic for another recipe.) Spoon the egg mixture onto each piece of toast and serve.

Per Serving

calories: 313 | fat: 10g | protein: 17g
carbs: 38g | fiber: 8g | sodium: 559mg

Feta and Pepper Frittata

Prep time: 10 minutes | Cook time: 20 minutes | Serves 4

Ingredients:

Olive oil cooking spray
8 large eggs
1 medium red bell pepper, diced
½ teaspoon salt
½ teaspoon black pepper
1 garlic clove, minced
½ cup feta, divided

Directions:

1. Preheat the air fryer to 360ºF (182ºC). Lightly coat the inside of a 6-inch round cake pan with olive oil cooking spray.
2. In a large bowl, beat the eggs for 1 to 2 minutes, or until well combined.
3. Add the bell pepper, salt, black pepper, and garlic to the eggs, and mix together until the bell pepper is distributed throughout.
4. Fold in ¼ cup of the feta cheese.
5. Pour the egg mixture into the prepared cake pan, and sprinkle the remaining ¼ cup of feta over the top.
6. Place into the air fryer and bake for 18 to 20 minutes, or until the eggs are set in the center.
7. Remove from the air fryer and allow to cool for 5 minutes before serving.

Per Serving

calories: 204 | fat: 14g | protein: 16g
carbs: 4g | fiber: 1g | sodium: 606mg

Sweet Potato Toast

Prep time: 5 minutes | Cook time: 15 minutes | Serves 4

Ingredients:

2 plum tomatoes, halved
6 tablespoons extra-virgin olive oil, divided
Salt and freshly ground black pepper, to taste
2 large sweet potatoes, sliced lengthwise
1 cup fresh spinach
8 medium asparagus, trimmed
4 large cooked eggs or egg substitute (poached, scrambled, or fried)
1 cup arugula
4 tablespoons pesto
4 tablespoons shredded Asiago cheese

Directions:

1. Preheat the oven to 450ºF (235ºC).
2. On a baking sheet, brush the plum tomato halves with 2 tablespoons of olive oil and season with salt and pepper. Roast the tomatoes in the oven for approximately 15 minutes, then remove from the oven and allow to rest.
3. Put the sweet potato slices on a separate baking sheet and brush about 2 tablespoons of oil on each side and season with salt and pepper. Bake the sweet potato slices for about 15 minutes, flipping once after 5 to 7 minutes, until just tender. Remove from the oven and set aside.
4. In a sauté pan or skillet, heat the remaining 2 tablespoons of olive oil over medium heat and sauté the fresh spinach until just wilted. Remove from the pan and rest on a paper towel-lined dish. In the same pan, add the asparagus and sauté, turning throughout. Transfer to a paper towel-lined dish.
5. Place the slices of grilled sweet potato on serving plates and divide the spinach and asparagus evenly among the slices. Place a prepared egg on top of the spinach and asparagus. Top this with ¼ cup of arugula.
6. Finish by drizzling with 1 tablespoon of pesto and sprinkle with 1 tablespoon of cheese. Serve with 1 roasted plum tomato.

Per Serving

calories: 441 | fat: 35g | protein: 13g
carbs: 23g | fiber: 4g | sodium: 481mg

Orange French Toast

Prep time: 5 minutes | Cook time: 15 minutes | Serves 6

Ingredients:

1 cup unsweetened almond milk
3 large eggs
2 teaspoons grated orange zest
1 teaspoon vanilla extract
⅛ teaspoon ground cardamom
⅛ teaspoon ground cinnamon
1 loaf of boule bread, sliced 1 inch thick (gluten-free preferred)
1 banana, sliced
¼ cup Berry and Honey Compote

Directions:

1. Heat a large nonstick sauté pan or skillet over medium-high heat.
2. In a large, shallow dish, mix the milk, eggs, orange zest, vanilla, cardamom, and cinnamon. Working in batches, dredge the bread slices in the egg mixture and put in the hot pan.
3. Cook for 5 minutes on each side, until golden brown. Serve, topped with banana and drizzled with honey compote.

Per Serving

calories: 394 | fat: 6g | protein: 17g
carbs: 68g | fiber: 3g | sodium: 716mg

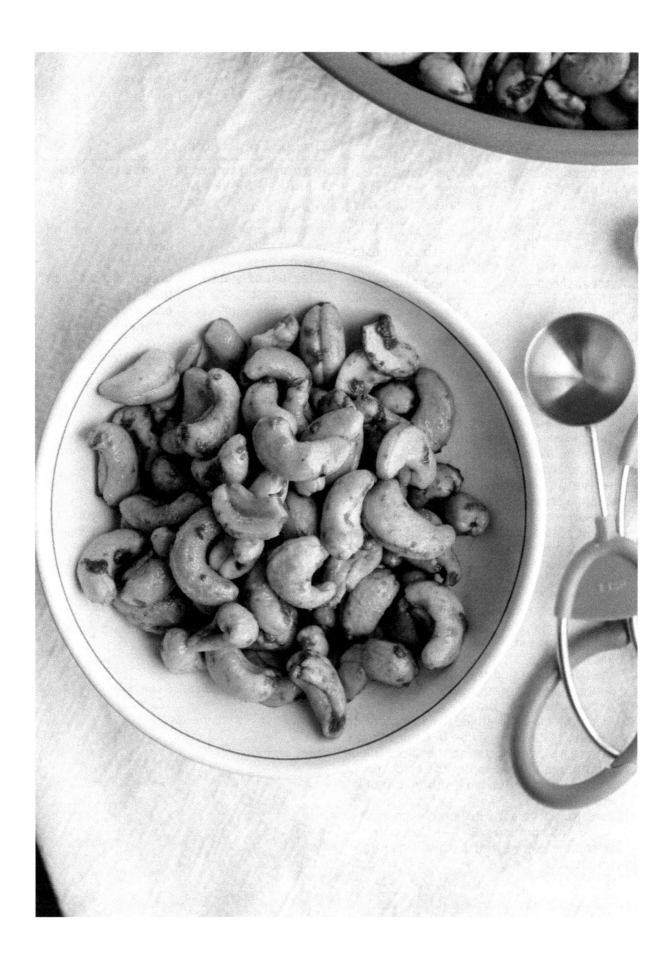

Chapter 2 Appetizers and Snacks

Pickled Turnips

Prep time: 5 minutes | Cook time: 0 minutes | Makes about 1 quart

Ingredients:

1 pound (454 g) turnips, washed well, peeled, and cut into 1-inch batons
1 small beet, roasted, peeled, and cut into 1-inch batons
2 garlic cloves, smashed
1 teaspoon dried Turkish oregano
3 cups warm water
½ cup red wine vinegar
½ cup white vinegar

Directions:

1. In a jar, combine the turnips, beet, garlic, and oregano. Pour the water and vinegars over the vegetables, cover, then shake well and put it in the refrigerator. The turnips will be pickled after 1 hour.

Per Serving (1 to 2 tablespoons)

calories: 8 | fat: 0g | protein: 1g
carbs: 1g | fiber: 0g | sodium: 6mg

Fried Halloumi with Tomato

Prep time: 2 minutes | Cook time: 5 minutes | Serves 2

Ingredients:

3 ounces (85 g) Halloumi cheese, cut crosswise into 2 thinner, rectangular pieces
2 teaspoons prepared pesto sauce, plus additional for drizzling
1 medium tomato, sliced

Directions:

1. Heat a nonstick skillet over medium-high heat and place the slices of Halloumi in the hot pan. After about 2 minutes, check to see if the cheese is golden on the bottom. If it is, flip the slices, top each with 1 teaspoon of pesto, and cook for another 2 minutes, or until the second side is golden.
2. Serve with slices of tomato and a drizzle of pesto, if desired, on the side.

Per Serving

calories: 177 | fat: 14g | protein: 10g
carbs: 4g | fiber: 1g | sodium: 233mg

Spiced Cashews

Prep time: 5 minutes | Cook time: 10 minutes | Serves 4

Ingredients:

2 cups raw cashews
2 tablespoons olive oil
¼ teaspoon salt
¼ teaspoon chili powder
⅛ teaspoon garlic powder
⅛ teaspoon smoked paprika

Directions:

1. Preheat the air fryer to 360ºF (182ºC).
2. In a large bowl, toss all of the ingredients together.
3. Pour the cashews into the air fryer basket and roast them for 5 minutes. Shake the basket, then cook for 5 minutes more.
4. Serve immediately.

Per Serving

calories: 476 | fat: 40g | protein: 14g
carbs: 23g | fiber: 3g | sodium: 151mg

Sweet Potato Chips

Prep time: 5 minutes | Cook time: 15 minutes | Serves 2

Ingredients:

1 large sweet potato, thinly sliced
⅛ teaspoon salt
2 tablespoons olive oil

Directions:

1. Preheat the air fryer to 380ºF (193ºC).
2. In a small bowl, toss the sweet potatoes, salt, and olive oil together until the potatoes are well coated.
3. Put the sweet potato slices into the air fryer and spread them out in a single layer.
4. Fry for 10 minutes. Stir, then air fry for 3 to 5 minutes more, or until the chips reach the preferred level of crispiness.

Per Serving

calories: 175 | fat: 14g | protein: 1g
carbs: 13g | fiber: 2g | sodium: 191mg

Kalamata Olive Tapenade

Prep time: 10 minutes | Cook time: 0 minutes | Makes 2 cups

Ingredients:

2 cups pitted Kalamata olives or other black olives
2 anchovy fillets, chopped
2 teaspoons chopped capers
1 garlic clove, finely minced
1 cooked egg yolk
1 teaspoon Dijon mustard
¼ cup extra-virgin olive oil
Vegetables, for serving (optional)

Directions:

1. Rinse the olives in cold water and drain well.
2. In a food processor, blender, or a large jar (if using an immersion blender) place the drained olives, anchovies, capers, garlic, egg yolk, and Dijon. Process until it forms a thick paste.
3. With the food processor running, slowly stream in the olive oil.
4. Transfer to a small bowl, cover, and refrigerate at least 1 hour to let the flavors develop. Serve with your favorite crunchy vegetables.

Per Serving (¹/₃ cup)

calories: 179 | fat: 19g | protein: 2g
carbs: 3g | fiber: 2g | sodium: 812mg

Caprese Stack with Burrata Cheese

Prep time: 5 minutes | Cook time: 0 minutes | Serves 4

Ingredients:

1 large organic tomato, preferably heirloom
½ teaspoon salt
¼ teaspoon freshly ground black pepper
1 (4-ounce / 113-g) ball burrata cheese
8 fresh basil leaves, thinly sliced
2 tablespoons extra-virgin olive oil
1 tablespoon red wine or balsamic vinegar

Directions:

1. Slice the tomato into 4 thick slices, removing any tough center core and sprinkle with salt and pepper. Place the tomatoes, seasoned-side up, on a plate.
2. On a separate rimmed plate, slice the burrata into 4 thick slices and place one slice on top of each tomato slice. Top each with one-quarter of the basil and pour any reserved burrata cream from the rimmed plate over top.
3. Drizzle with olive oil and vinegar and serve with a fork and knife.

Per Serving (1 stack)

calories: 153 | fat: 13g | protein: 7g
carbs: 2g | fiber: 1g | sodium: 469mg

Cranberry Chocolate Granola Bars

Prep time: 5 minutes | Cook time: 15 minutes | Serves 6

Ingredients:

2 cups certified gluten-free quick oats
2 tablespoons sugar-free dark chocolate chunks
2 tablespoons unsweetened dried cranberries
3 tablespoons unsweetened shredded coconut
½ cup raw honey
1 teaspoon ground cinnamon
⅛ teaspoon salt
2 tablespoons olive oil

Directions:

1. Preheat the air fryer to 360ºF (182ºC). Line an 8-by-8-inch baking dish with parchment paper that comes up the side so you can lift it out after cooking.
2. In a large bowl, mix together all of the ingredients until well combined.
3. Press the oat mixture into the pan in an even layer.
4. Place the pan into the air fryer basket and bake for 15 minutes.
5. Remove the pan from the air fryer, and lift the granola cake out of the pan using the edges of the parchment paper.
6. Allow to cool for 5 minutes before slicing into 6 equal bars.
7. Serve immediately, or wrap in plastic wrap and store at room temperature for up to 1 week.

Per Serving

calories: 272 | fat: 10g | protein: 6g
carbs: 55g | fiber: 5g | sodium: 74mg

Salmon and Avocado Stuffed Cucumbers

Prep time: 10 minutes | Cook time: 0 minutes | Serves 4

Ingredients:

2 large cucumbers, peeled
1 (4-ounce / 113-g) can red salmon
1 medium very ripe avocado, peeled, pitted, and mashed
1 tablespoon extra-virgin olive oil

Zest and juice of 1 lime
3 tablespoons chopped fresh cilantro
½ teaspoon salt
¼ teaspoon freshly ground black pepper

Directions:

1. Slice the cucumber into 1-inch-thick segments and using a spoon, scrape seeds out of center of each segment and stand up on a plate.
2. In a medium bowl, combine the salmon, avocado, olive oil, lime zest and juice, cilantro, salt, and pepper and mix until creamy.
3. Spoon the salmon mixture into the center of each cucumber segment and serve chilled.

Per Serving

calories: 159 | fat: 11g | protein: 9g
carbs: 8g | fiber: 3g | sodium: 398mg

Mackerel Pâté with Horseradish

Prep time: 10 minutes | Cook time: 0 minutes | Serves 4

Ingredients:

4 ounces (113 g) olive oil-packed wild-caught mackerel
2 ounces (57 g) goat cheese
Zest and juice of 1 lemon
2 tablespoons chopped fresh parsley
2 tablespoons chopped fresh

arugula
1 tablespoon extra-virgin olive oil
2 teaspoons chopped capers
1 to 2 teaspoons fresh horseradish (optional)
Crackers, cucumber rounds, endive spears, or celery, for serving (optional)

Directions:

1. In a food processor, blender, or large bowl with immersion blender, combine the mackerel, goat cheese, lemon zest and juice, parsley, arugula, olive oil, capers, and horseradish (if using). Process or blend until smooth and creamy.
2. Serve with crackers, cucumber rounds, endive spears, or celery.
3. Store covered in the refrigerator for up to 1 week.

Per Serving

calories: 118 | fat: 8g | protein: 9g
carbs: 1g | fiber: 0g | sodium: 196mg

Lemon Marinated Feta and Artichokes

Prep time: 10 minutes | Cook time: 0 minutes | Makes 1½ cups

Ingredients:

4 ounces (113 g) traditional Greek feta, cut into ½-inch cubes
4 ounces (113 g) drained artichoke hearts, quartered lengthwise
⅓ cup extra-virgin olive oil

Zest and juice of 1 lemon
2 tablespoons roughly chopped fresh rosemary
2 tablespoons roughly chopped fresh parsley
½ teaspoon black peppercorns

Directions:

1. In a glass bowl or large glass jar, combine the feta and artichoke hearts. Add the olive oil, lemon zest and juice, rosemary, parsley, and peppercorns and toss gently to coat, being sure not to crumble the feta.
2. Cover and refrigerate for at least 4 hours, or up to 4 days. Pull out of the refrigerator 30 minutes before serving.

Per Serving (⅓ cup)

calories: 235 | fat: 23g | protein: 4g
carbs: 3g | fiber: 1g | sodium: 406mg

Falafel Balls with Garlic-Yogurt Sauce

Prep time: 5 minutes | Cook time: 15 minutes | Serves 4

Ingredients:

Falafel:

1 (15-ounce / 425-g) can chickpeas, drained and rinsed
½ cup fresh parsley
2 garlic cloves, minced

½ tablespoon ground cumin
1 tablespoon whole wheat flour
Salt, to taste

Garlic-Yogurt Sauce:

1 cup nonfat plain Greek yogurt
1 garlic clove, minced

1 tablespoon chopped fresh dill
2 tablespoons lemon juice

Directions:

Make the Falafel

1. Preheat the air fryer to 360ºF (182ºC).
2. Put the chickpeas into a food processor. Pulse until mostly chopped, then add the parsley, garlic, and cumin and pulse for another 1 to 2 minutes, or until the ingredients are combined and turning into a dough.
3. Add the flour. Pulse a few more times until combined. The dough will have texture, but the chickpeas should be pulsed into small bits.
4. Using clean hands, roll the dough into 8 balls of equal size, then pat the balls down a bit so they are about ½-thick disks.
5. Spray the basket of the air fryer with olive oil cooking spray, then place the falafel patties in the basket in a single layer, making sure they don't touch each other.
6. Fry in the air fryer for 15 minutes.

Make the Garlic-Yogurt Sauce

7. In a small bowl, combine the yogurt, garlic, dill, and lemon juice.
8. Once the falafel are done cooking and nicely browned on all sides, remove them from the air fryer and season with salt.
9. Serve hot with a side of dipping sauce.

Per Serving

calories: 151 | fat: 2g | protein: 12g
carbs: 22g | fiber: 5g | sodium: 141mg

Fried Green Beans

Prep time: 5 minutes | Cook time: 5 minutes | Serves 4

Ingredients:

Green Beans:

1 egg
2 tablespoons water
1 tablespoon whole wheat flour
¼ teaspoon paprika
½ teaspoon garlic

powder
½ teaspoon salt
¼ cup whole wheat bread crumbs
½ pound (227 g) whole green beans

Lemon-Yogurt Sauce:

½ cup nonfat plain Greek yogurt
1 tablespoon lemon juice

¼ teaspoon salt
⅛ teaspoon cayenne pepper

Directions:

1. Preheat the air fryer to 380ºF (193ºC).
2. In a medium shallow bowl, beat together the egg and water until frothy.
3. In a separate medium shallow bowl, whisk together the flour, paprika, garlic powder, and salt, then mix in the bread crumbs.
4. Spray the bottom of the air fryer with cooking spray.
5. Dip each green bean into the egg mixture, then into the bread crumb mixture, coating the outside with the crumbs. Place the green beans in a single layer in the bottom of the air fryer basket.
6. Fry in the air fryer for 5 minutes, or until the breading is golden brown.
7. Make the Lemon-Yogurt Sauce
8. In a small bowl, combine the yogurt, lemon juice, salt, and cayenne.
9. Serve the green bean fries alongside the lemon-yogurt sauce as a snack or appetizer.

Per Serving

calories: 88 | fat: 2g | protein: 7g
carbs: 12g | fiber: 2g | sodium: 502mg

Whole Wheat Pita Chips

Prep time: 2 minutes | Cook time: 8 minutes | Serves 2

Ingredients:

2 whole wheat pitas
1 tablespoon olive oil
½ teaspoon kosher salt

Directions:

1. Preheat the air fryer to 360ºF (182ºC).
2. Cut each pita into 8 wedges.
3. In a medium bowl, toss the pita wedges, olive oil, and salt until the wedges are coated and the olive oil and salt are evenly distributed.
4. Place the pita wedges into the air fryer basket in an even layer and fry for 6 to 8 minutes. (The cooking time will vary depending upon how thick the pita is and how browned you prefer a chip.)
5. Season with additional salt, if desired. Serve alone or with a favorite dip.

Per Serving

calories: 230 | fat: 8g | protein: 6g
carbs: 35g | fiber: 4g | sodium: 706mg

Greek-Style Potato Skins

Prep time: 5 minutes | Cook time: 45 minutes | Serves 4

Ingredients:

2 russet potatoes
3 tablespoons olive oil, divided, plus more for drizzling (optional)
1 teaspoon kosher salt, divided
¼ teaspoon black pepper
2 tablespoons fresh cilantro, chopped, plus more for serving
¼ cup Kalamata olives, diced
¼ cup crumbled feta
Chopped fresh parsley, for garnish (optional)

Directions:

1. Preheat the air fryer to 380ºF (193ºC).
2. Using a fork, poke 2 to 3 holes in the potatoes, then coat each with about ½ tablespoon olive oil and ½ teaspoon salt.
3. Place the potatoes into the air fryer basket and bake for 30 minutes.
4. Remove the potatoes from the air fryer, and slice in half. Using a spoon, scoop out the flesh of the potatoes, leaving a ½-inch layer of potato inside the skins, and set the skins aside.
5. In a medium bowl, combine the scooped potato middles with the remaining 2 tablespoons of olive oil, ½ teaspoon of salt, black pepper, and cilantro. Mix until well combined.
6. Divide the potato filling into the now-empty potato skins, spreading it evenly over them. Top each potato with a tablespoon each of the olives and feta.
7. Place the loaded potato skins back into the air fryer and bake for 15 minutes.
8. Serve with additional chopped cilantro or parsley and a drizzle of olive oil, if desired.

Per Serving

calories: 270 | fat: 13g | protein: 5g
carbs: 34g | fiber: 3g | sodium: 748mg

Creamy Hummus

Prep time: 5 minutes | Cook time: 0 minutes | Serves 8

Ingredients:

1 (15-ounce / 425-g) can garbanzo beans, rinsed and drained
2 cloves garlic, peeled
¼ cup lemon juice
1 teaspoon salt
¼ cup plain Greek yogurt
½ cup tahini paste
2 tablespoons extra-virgin olive oil, divided

Directions:

1. Add the garbanzo beans, garlic cloves, lemon juice, and salt to a food processor fitted with a chopping blade. Blend for 1 minute, until smooth.
2. Scrape down the sides of the processor. Add the Greek yogurt, tahini paste, and 1 tablespoon of olive oil and blend for another minute, until creamy and well combined.
3. Spoon the hummus into a serving bowl. Drizzle the remaining tablespoon of olive oil on top.

Per Serving

calories: 189 | fat: 13g | protein: 7g
carbs: 14g | fiber: 4g | sodium: 313mg

Healthy Deviled Eggs with Greek Yogurt

Prep time: 15 minutes | Cook time: 15 minutes | Serves 4

Ingredients:

4 eggs
¼ cup nonfat plain Greek yogurt
1 teaspoon chopped fresh dill
⅛ teaspoon salt
⅛ teaspoon paprika
⅛ teaspoon garlic powder
Chopped fresh parsley, for garnish

Directions:

1. Preheat the air fryer to 270ºF (132ºC).
2. Place the eggs in a single layer in the air fryer basket and cook for 15 min.
3. Quickly remove the eggs from the air fryer and place them into a cold water
4. bath. Let the eggs cool in the water for 10 minutes before removing and
5. peeling them.
6. After peeling the eggs, cut them in half.
7. Spoon the yolk into a small bowl. Add the yogurt, dill, salt, paprika, and garlic
8. powder and mix until smooth.
9. Spoon or pipe the yolk mixture into the halved egg whites. Serve with a
10. sprinkle of fresh parsley on top.

Per Serving

calories: 80 | fat: 5g | protein: 8g
carbs: 1g | fiber: 0g | sodium: 149mg

Tuna and Caper Croquettes

Prep time: 10 minutes | Cook time: 25 minutes | Makes 36 croquettes

Ingredients:

6 tablespoons extra-virgin olive oil, plus 1 to 2 cups
5 tablespoons almond flour, plus 1 cup, divided
1¼ cups heavy cream
1 (4-ounce / 113-g) can olive oil-packed yellowfin tuna
1 tablespoon chopped red onion
2 teaspoons minced capers
½ teaspoon dried dill
¼ teaspoon freshly ground black pepper
2 large eggs
1 cup panko bread crumbs (or a gluten-free version)

Directions:

1. In a large skillet, heat 6 tablespoons olive oil over medium-low heat. Add 5 tablespoons almond flour and cook, stirring constantly, until a smooth paste forms and the flour browns slightly, 2 to 3 minutes.
2. Increase the heat to medium-high and gradually add the heavy cream, whisking constantly until completely smooth and thickened, another 4 to 5 minutes.
3. Remove from the heat and stir in the tuna, red onion, capers, dill, and pepper.
4. Transfer the mixture to an 8-inch square baking dish that is well coated with olive oil and allow to cool to room temperature. Cover and refrigerate until chilled, at least 4 hours or up to overnight.
5. To form the croquettes, set out three bowls. In one, beat together the eggs. In another, add the remaining almond flour. In the third, add the panko. Line a baking sheet with parchment paper.
6. Using a spoon, place about a tablespoon of cold prepared dough into the flour mixture and roll to coat. Shake off excess and, using your hands, roll into an oval.
7. Dip the croquette into the beaten egg, then lightly coat in panko. Set on lined baking sheet and repeat with the remaining dough.
8. In a small saucepan, heat the remaining 1 to 2 cups of olive oil, so that the oil is about 1 inch deep, over medium-high heat. The smaller the pan, the less oil you will need, but you will need more for each batch.
9. Test if the oil is ready by throwing a pinch of panko into pot. If it sizzles, the oil is ready for frying. If it sinks, it's not quite ready. Once the oil is heated, fry the croquettes 3 or 4 at a time, depending on the size of your pan, removing with a slotted spoon when golden brown. You will need to adjust the temperature of the oil occasionally to prevent burning. If the croquettes get dark brown very quickly, lower the temperature.

Per Serving (3 croquettes)

calories: 245 | fat: 22g | protein: 6g
carbs: 7g | fiber: 1g | sodium: 85mg

Beet Chips

Prep time: 10 minutes | Cook time: 30 minutes | Serves 6

Ingredients:

4 medium beets, rinse and thinly sliced
1 teaspoon sea salt
2 tablespoons olive oil
Hummus, for serving

Directions:

1. Preheat the air fryer to 380ºF (193ºC).
2. In a large bowl, toss the beets with sea salt and olive oil until well coated.
3. Put the beet slices into the air fryer and spread them out in a single layer.
4. Fry for 10 minutes. Stir, then fry for an additional 10 minutes. Stir again,
5. then fry for a final 5 to 10 minutes, or until the chips reach the desired crispiness.
6. Serve with a favorite hummus.

Per Serving

calories: 63 | fat: 5g | protein: 1g
carbs: 5g | fiber: 2g | sodium: 430mg

Quinoa-Feta Stuffed Mushrooms

Prep time: 5 minutes | Cook time: 8 minutes | Serves 6

Ingredients:

2 tablespoons finely diced red bell pepper
1 garlic clove, minced
¼ cup cooked quinoa
⅛ teaspoon salt
¼ teaspoon dried oregano
24 button mushrooms, stemmed
2 ounces (57 g) crumbled feta
3 tablespoons whole wheat bread crumbs
Olive oil cooking spray

Directions:

1. Preheat the air fryer to 360ºF (182ºC).
2. In a small bowl, combine the bell pepper, garlic, quinoa, salt, and oregano.
3. Spoon the quinoa stuffing into the mushroom caps until just filled.
4. Add a small piece of feta to the top of each mushroom.
5. Sprinkle a pinch bread crumbs over the feta on each mushroom.

6. Spray the basket of the air fryer with olive oil cooking spray, then gently place the mushrooms into the basket, making sure that they don't touch each other. (Depending on the size of the air fryer, you may have to cook them in two batches.)
7. Place the basket into the air fryer and bake for 8 minutes.
8. Remove from the air fryer and serve.

Per Serving (4 mushrooms)

calories: 97 | fat: 4g | protein: 7g
carbs: 11g | fiber: 2g | sodium: 167mg

Strawberry Caprese Skewers with Balsamic Glaze

Prep time: 15 minutes | Cook time: 10 minutes | Serves 2

Ingredients:

½ cup balsamic vinegar
16 whole, hulled strawberries
12 small basil leaves
or 6 large leaves, halved
12 pieces of small Mozzarella balls

Directions:

1. To make the balsamic glaze, pour the balsamic vinegar into a small saucepan and bring it to a boil. Reduce the heat to medium-low and simmer for 10 minutes, or until it's reduced by half and is thick enough to coat the back of a spoon.
2. On each of 4 wooden skewers, place a strawberry, a folded basil leaf, and a Mozzarella ball, repeating twice and adding a strawberry on the end. (Each skewer should have 4 strawberries, 3 basil leaves, and 3 Mozzarella balls.)
3. Drizzle 1 to 2 teaspoons of balsamic glaze over the skewers.

Per Serving

calories: 206 | fat: 10g | protein: 10g
carbs: 17g | fiber: 1g | sodium: 282mg

Citrus Garlic Marinated Olives

Prep time: 10 minutes | Cook time: 0 minutes | Makes 2 cups

Ingredients:

2 cups mixed green olives with pits
¼ cup red wine vinegar
¼ cup extra-virgin olive oil
4 garlic cloves, finely minced
Zest and juice of

2 clementines or 1 large orange
1 teaspoon red pepper flakes
2 bay leaves
½ teaspoon ground cumin
½ teaspoon ground allspice

Directions:

1. In a large glass bowl or jar, combine the olives, vinegar, oil, garlic, orange zest and juice, red pepper flakes, bay leaves, cumin, and allspice and mix well. Cover and refrigerate for at least 4 hours or up to a week to allow the olives to marinate, tossing again before serving.

Per Serving (¼ cup)

calories: 133 | fat: 14g | protein: 1g
carbs: 3g | fiber: 2g | sodium: 501mg

Homemade Trail Mix

Prep time: 10 minutes | Cook time: 10 minutes | Makes 4 cups

Ingredients:

1 tablespoon olive oil
1 tablespoon maple syrup
1 teaspoon vanilla
½ teaspoon cardamom
½ teaspoon allspice
2 cups mixed, unsalted nuts

¼ cup unsalted pumpkin or sunflower seeds
½ cup dried apricots, diced or thinly sliced
½ cup dried figs, diced or thinly sliced
Pinch salt

Directions:

1. Combine the olive oil, maple syrup, vanilla, cardamom, and allspice in a large sauté pan over medium heat. Stir to combine.
2. Add the nuts and seeds and stir well to coat. Let the nuts and seeds toast for about 10 minutes, stirring frequently.

3. Remove from the heat, and add the dried apricots and figs. Stir everything well and season with salt.
4. Store in an airtight container.

Per Serving (½ cup)

calories: 261 | fat: 18g | protein: 6g
carbs: 23g | fiber: 5g | sodium: 26mg

Labneh Vegetable Parfaits

Prep time: 15 minutes | Cook time: 0 minutes | Serves 2

Ingredients:

Labneh:

8 ounces (227 g) plain Greek yogurt (full-fat works best)
Generous pinch salt
1 teaspoon za'atar

seasoning
1 teaspoon freshly squeezed lemon juice
Pinch lemon zest

Parfaits:

½ cup peeled, chopped cucumber
½ cup grated carrots

½ cup cherry tomatoes, halved

Directions:

Make the Labneh

1. Line a strainer with cheesecloth and place it over a bowl.
2. Stir together the Greek yogurt and salt and place in the cheesecloth. Wrap it up and let it sit for 24 hours in the refrigerator.
3. When ready, unwrap the labneh and place it into a clean bowl. Stir in the za'atar, lemon juice, and lemon zest.

Make the Parfaits

4. Divide the cucumber between two clear glasses.
5. Top each portion of cucumber with about 3 tablespoons of labneh.
6. Divide the carrots between the glasses.
7. Top with another 3 tablespoons of the labneh.
8. Top parfaits with the cherry tomatoes.

Per Serving

calories: 143 | fat: 7g | protein: 5g
carbs: 16g | fiber: 2g | sodium: 187mg

Rosemary and Honey Almonds

Prep time: 5 minutes | Cook time: 10 minutes | Serves 6

Ingredients:

1 cup raw, whole, shelled almonds
1 tablespoon minced fresh rosemary
¼ teaspoon kosher or sea salt
1 tablespoon honey
Nonstick cooking spray

Directions:

1. In a large skillet over medium heat, combine the almonds, rosemary, and salt. Stir frequently for 1 minute.
2. Drizzle in the honey and cook for another 3 to 4 minutes, stirring frequently, until the almonds are coated and just starting to darken around the edges.
3. Remove from the heat. Using a spatula, spread the almonds onto a pan coated with nonstick cooking spray. Cool for 10 minutes or so. Break up the almonds before serving.

Per Serving

calories: 13 | fat: 1g | protein: 1g
carbs: 3g | fiber: 1g | sodium: 97mg

Crunchy Chili Chickpeas

Prep time: 5 minutes | Cook time: 15 minutes | Serves 4

Ingredients:

1 (15-ounce / 425-g) can cooked chickpeas, drained and rinsed
1 tablespoon olive oil
¼ teaspoon salt
⅛ teaspoon chili powder
⅛ teaspoon garlic powder
⅛ teaspoon paprika

Directions:

1. Preheat the air fryer to 380ºF (193ºC).
2. In a medium bowl, toss all of the ingredients together until the chickpeas are well coated.
3. Pour the chickpeas into the air fryer and spread them out in a single layer.
4. Roast for 15 minutes, stirring once halfway through the cook time.

Per Serving

calories: 109 | fat: 5g | protein: 4g
carbs: 13g | fiber: 4g | sodium: 283mg

Spiced Roasted Chickpeas

Prep time: 15 minutes | Cook time: 35 minutes | Serves 2

Ingredients:

Seasoning Mix:

¾ teaspoon cumin
½ teaspoon coriander
½ teaspoon salt
¼ teaspoon freshly ground black pepper
¼ teaspoon paprika
¼ teaspoon cardamom
¼ teaspoon cinnamon
¼ teaspoon allspice

Chickpeas:

1 (15-ounce / 425-g) can chickpeas, drained and rinsed
1 tablespoon olive oil
¼ teaspoon salt

Directions:

Make the Seasoning Mix

1. In a small bowl, combine the cumin, coriander, salt, freshly ground black pepper, paprika, cardamom, cinnamon, and allspice. Stir well to combine and set aside.

Make the Chickpeas

2. Preheat the oven to 400ºF (205ºC) and set the rack to the middle position. Line a baking sheet with parchment paper.
3. Pat the rinsed chickpeas with paper towels or roll them in a clean kitchen towel to dry off any water.
4. Place the chickpeas in a bowl and season them with the olive oil and salt.
5. Add the chickpeas to the lined baking sheet (reserve the bowl) and roast them for about 25 to 35 minutes, turning them over once or twice while cooking. Most should be light brown. Taste one or two to make sure they are slightly crisp.
6. Place the roasted chickpeas back into the bowl and sprinkle them with the seasoning mix. Toss lightly to combine. Taste, and add additional salt if needed. Serve warm.

Per Serving

calories: 268 | fat: 11g | protein: 11g
carbs: 35g | fiber: 10g | sodium: 301mg

Roasted Figs with Goat Cheese

Prep time: 5 minutes | Cook time: 10 minutes | Serves 4

Ingredients:

8 fresh figs
2 ounces (57 g) goat cheese
¼ teaspoon ground
cinnamon
1 tablespoon honey, plus more for serving
1 tablespoon olive oil

Directions:

1. Preheat the air fryer to 360ºF (182ºC).
2. Cut the stem off of each fig.
3. Cut an X into the top of each fig, cutting halfway down the fig. Leave the base intact.
4. In a small bowl, mix together the goat cheese, cinnamon, and honey.
5. Spoon the goat cheese mixture into the cavity of each fig.
6. Place the figs in a single layer in the air fryer basket. Drizzle the olive oil over top of the figs and roast for 10 minutes.
7. Serve with an additional drizzle of honey.

Per Serving

calories: 158 | fat: 7g | protein: 3g
carbs: 24g | fiber: 3g | sodium: 61mg

Carrot Cake Cupcakes with Walnuts

Prep time: 10 minutes | Cook time: 12 minutes | Serves 6

Ingredients:

Olive oil cooking spray
1 cup grated carrots
¼ cup raw honey
¼ cup olive oil
½ teaspoon vanilla extract
1 egg
¼ cup unsweetened applesauce
1 ⅓ cups whole wheat flour
¾ teaspoon baking powder
½ teaspoon baking soda
½ teaspoon ground cinnamon
¼ teaspoon ground nutmeg
⅛ teaspoon ground ginger
⅛ teaspoon salt
¼ cup chopped walnuts
2 tablespoons chopped golden raisins

Directions:

1. Preheat the air fryer to 380ºF (193ºC). Lightly coat the inside of six silicone muffin cups or a six-cup muffin tin with olive oil cooking spray.
2. In a medium bowl, mix together the carrots, honey, olive oil, vanilla extract, egg, and unsweetened applesauce.
3. In a separate medium bowl, whisk together the flour, baking powder, baking soda, cinnamon, nutmeg, ginger, and salt.
4. Add the wet ingredients to the dry ingredients, mixing until just combined.
5. Gently fold in the walnuts and raisins. Fill the muffin cups or tin three-quarters full with the batter, and place them in the air fryer basket.
6. Bake for 10 to 12 minutes, or until a toothpick inserted in the center of a cupcake comes out clean.
7. Serve immediately or store in an airtight container until ready to serve.

Per Serving

calories: 277 | fat: 14g | protein: 6g
carbs: 36g | fiber: 4g | sodium: 182mg

Garlic and Herb Marinated Artichokes

Prep time: 10 minutes | Cook time: 0 minutes | Makes 2 cups

Ingredients:

2 (13¾-ounce / 390-g) cans artichoke hearts, drained and quartered
¾ cup extra-virgin olive oil
4 small garlic cloves, crushed with the back of a knife
1 tablespoon fresh
rosemary leaves
2 teaspoons chopped fresh oregano or
1 teaspoon dried oregano
1 teaspoon red pepper flakes (optional)
1 teaspoon salt

Directions:

1. In a medium bowl, combine the artichoke hearts, olive oil, garlic, rosemary, oregano, red pepper flakes (if using), and salt. Toss to combine well.
2. Store in an airtight glass container in the refrigerator and marinate for at least 24 hours before using. Store in the refrigerator for up to 2 weeks.

Per Serving (¼ cup)

calories: 275 | fat: 27g | protein: 4g
carbs: 11g | fiber: 4g | sodium: 652mg

Cucumber Cup Appetizers

Prep time: 5 minutes | Cook time: 0 minutes | Serves 2

Ingredients:

1 medium cucumber (about 8 ounces / 227 g, 8 to 9 inches long)
½ cup hummus (any flavor) or white bean dip
4 or 5 cherry tomatoes, sliced in half
2 tablespoons fresh basil, minced

Directions:

1. Slice the ends off the cucumber (about ½ inch from each side) and slice the cucumber into 1-inch pieces.
2. With a paring knife or a spoon, scoop most of the seeds from the inside of each cucumber piece to make a cup, being careful to not cut all the way through.
3. Fill each cucumber cup with about 1 tablespoon of hummus or bean dip.
4. Top each with a cherry tomato half and a sprinkle of fresh minced basil.

Per Serving

calories: 135 | fat: 6g | protein: 6g
carbs: 16g | fiber: 5g | sodium: 242mg

Apple Chips with Chocolate Tahini Sauce

Prep time: 10 minutes | Cook time: 0 minutes | Serves 2

Ingredients:

2 tablespoons tahini
1 tablespoon maple syrup
1 tablespoon unsweetened cocoa powder
1 to 2 tablespoons
warm water (or more if needed)
2 medium apples
1 tablespoon roasted, salted sunflower seeds

Directions:

1. In a small bowl, mix together the tahini, maple syrup, and cocoa powder. Add warm water, a little at a time, until thin enough to drizzle. Do not microwave it to thin it—it won't work.
2. Slice the apples crosswise into round slices, and then cut each piece in half to make a chip.
3. Lay the apple chips out on a plate and drizzle them with the chocolate tahini sauce.
4. Sprinkle sunflower seeds over the apple chips.

Per Serving

calories: 261 | fat: 11g | protein: 5g
carbs: 43g | fiber: 8g | sodium: 21mg

Mediterranean White Beans with Basil

Prep time: 2 minutes | Cook time: 19 minutes | Serves 2

Ingredients:

1 (15-ounce / 425-g) can cooked white beans
2 tablespoons olive oil
1 teaspoon fresh sage, chopped
¼ teaspoon garlic powder
¼ teaspoon salt, divided
1 teaspoon chopped fresh basil

Directions:

1. Preheat the air fryer to 380ºF (193ºC).
2. In a medium bowl, mix together the beans, olive oil, sage, garlic, ⅛ teaspoon
3. salt, and basil.
4. Pour the white beans into the air fryer and spread them out in a single layer.
5. Bake for 10 minutes. Stir and continue cooking for an additional 5 to 9
6. minutes, or until they reach your preferred level of crispiness.
7. Toss with the remaining ⅛ teaspoon salt before serving.

Per Serving

calories: 308 | fat: 14g | protein: 13g
carbs: 34g | fiber: 9g | sodium: 294mg

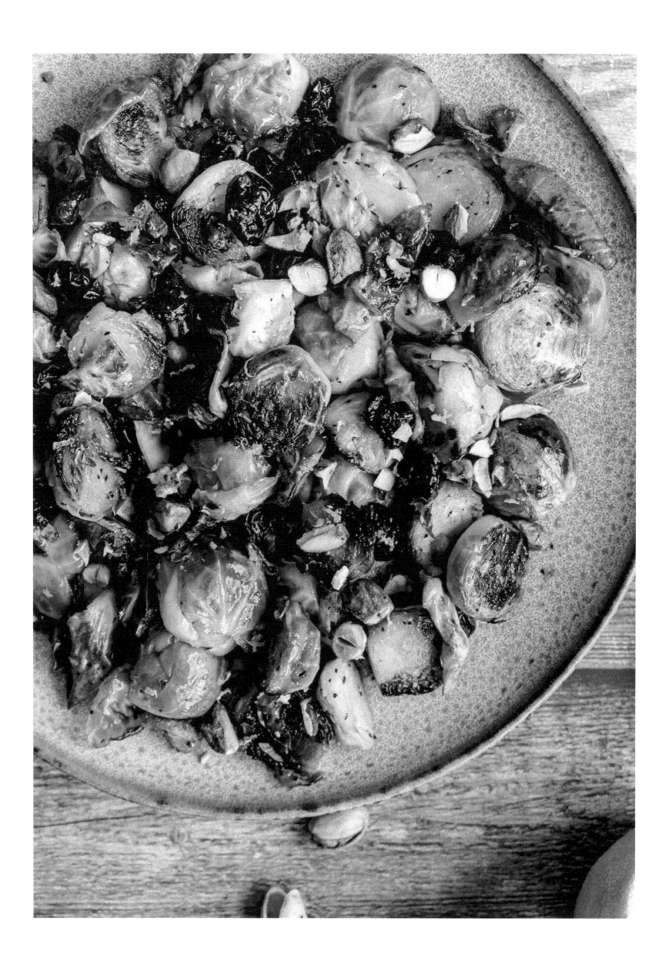

Chapter 3 Vegetables

Zucchini with Garlic and Red Pepper

Prep time: 5 minutes | Cook time: 15 minutes | Serves 6

Ingredients:

2 medium zucchini, cubed
1 red bell pepper, diced
2 garlic cloves, sliced
2 tablespoons olive oil
½ teaspoon salt

Directions:

1. Preheat the air fryer to 380ºF (193ºC).
2. In a large bowl, mix together the zucchini, bell pepper, and garlic with the olive oil and salt.
3. Pour the mixture into the air fryer basket, and roast for 7 minutes. Shake or stir, then roast for 7 to 8 minutes more.

Per Serving

calories: 60 | fat: 5g | protein: 1g
carbs: 4g | fiber: 1g | sodium: 195mg

Savory Sweet Potatoes with Parmesan

Prep time: 10 minutes | Cook time: 18 minutes | Serves 4

Ingredients:

2 large sweet potatoes, peeled and cubed
¼ cup olive oil
1 teaspoon dried
rosemary
½ teaspoon salt
2 tablespoons shredded Parmesan

Directions:

1. Preheat the air fryer to 360ºF (182ºC).
2. In a large bowl, toss the sweet potatoes with the olive oil, rosemary, and salt.
3. Pour the potatoes into the air fryer basket and roast for 10 minutes, then stir the potatoes and sprinkle the Parmesan over the top. Continue roasting for 8 minutes more.
4. Serve hot and enjoy.

Per Serving

calories: 186 | fat: 14g | protein: 2g
carbs: 13g | fiber: 2g | sodium: 369mg

Roasted Asparagus and Tomatoes

Prep time: 5 minutes | Cook time: 12 minutes | Serves 6

Ingredients:

2 cups grape tomatoes
1 bunch asparagus, trimmed
2 tablespoons olive
oil
3 garlic cloves, minced
½ teaspoon kosher salt

Directions:

1. Preheat the air fryer to 380ºF (193ºC).
2. In a large bowl, combine all of the ingredients, tossing until the vegetables are well coated with oil.
3. Pour the vegetable mixture into the air fryer basket and spread into a single layer, then roast for 12 minutes.

Per Serving

calories: 57 | fat: 5g | protein: 1g
carbs: 4g | fiber: 1g | sodium: 197mg

Orange Roasted Brussels Sprouts

Prep time: 5 minutes | Cook time: 10 minutes | Serves 4

Ingredients:

1 pound (454 g) Brussels sprouts, quartered
2 garlic cloves, minced
2 tablespoons olive oil
½ teaspoon salt
1 orange, cut into rings

Directions:

1. Preheat the air fryer to 360ºF (182ºC).
2. In a large bowl, toss the quartered Brussels sprouts with the garlic, olive oil, and salt until well coated.
3. Pour the Brussels sprouts into the air fryer, lay the orange slices on top of them, and roast for 10 minutes.
4. Remove from the air fryer and set the orange slices aside. Toss the Brussels sprouts before serving.

Per Serving

calories: 111 | fat: 7g | protein: 4g
carbs: 11g | fiber: 4g | sodium: 319mg

Traditional Moussaka

Prep time: 20 minutes | Cook time: 40 minutes | Serves 6

Ingredients:

2 large eggplants
2 teaspoons salt, divided
Olive oil spray, or olive oil for brushing
¼ cup extra-virgin olive oil
2 large onions, sliced
10 cloves garlic, sliced
2 (15-ounce / 425-g) cans diced tomatoes
1 (16-ounce / 454-g) can garbanzo beans, rinsed and drained
1 teaspoon dried oregano
½ teaspoon freshly ground black pepper

Directions:

1. Slice the eggplant horizontally into ¼-inch-thick round disks. Sprinkle the eggplant slices with 1 teaspoon of salt and place in a colander for 30 minutes. This will draw out the excess water from the eggplant.
2. Preheat the oven to 450ºF (235ºC). Pat the slices of eggplant dry with a paper towel and spray each side with an olive oil spray or lightly brush each side with olive oil.
3. Arrange the eggplant in a single layer on a baking sheet. Put in the oven and bake for 10 minutes. Then, using a spatula, flip the slices over and bake for another 10 minutes.
4. In a large skillet add the olive oil, onions, garlic, and remaining 1 teaspoon of salt. Cook for 3 to 5 minutes stirring occasionally. Add the tomatoes, garbanzo beans, oregano, and black pepper. Simmer for 10 to 12 minutes, stirring occasionally.
5. Using a deep casserole dish, begin to layer, starting with eggplant, then the sauce. Repeat until all ingredients have been used. Bake in the oven for 20 minutes.
6. Remove from the oven and serve warm.

Per Serving

calories: 262 | fat: 11g | protein: 8g
carbs: 35g | fiber: 11g | sodium: 1043mg

Rosemary Roasted Red Potatoes

Prep time: 5 minutes | Cook time: 20 minutes | Serves 6

Ingredients:

1 pound (454 g) red potatoes, quartered
¼ cup olive oil
½ teaspoon kosher salt
¼ teaspoon black pepper
1 garlic clove, minced
4 rosemary sprigs

Directions:

1. Preheat the air fryer to 360ºF (182ºC).
2. In a large bowl, toss the potatoes with the olive oil, salt, pepper, and garlic until well coated.
3. Pour the potatoes into the air fryer basket and top with the sprigs of rosemary.
4. Roast for 10 minutes, then stir or toss the potatoes and roast for 10 minutes more.
5. Remove the rosemary sprigs and serve the potatoes. Season with additional salt and pepper, if needed.

Per Serving

calories: 133 | fat: 9g | protein: 1g
carbs: 12g | fiber: 1g | sodium: 199mg

Easy Roasted Radishes

Prep time: 5 minutes | Cook time: 18 minutes | Serves 4

Ingredients:

1 pound (454 g) radishes, ends trimmed if needed
2 tablespoons olive oil
½ teaspoon sea salt

Directions:

1. Preheat the air fryer to 360ºF (182ºC).
2. In a large bowl, combine the radishes with olive oil and sea salt.
3. Pour the radishes into the air fryer and cook for 10 minutes. Stir or turn the radishes over and cook for 8 minutes more, then serve.

Per Serving

calories: 78 | fat: 9g | protein: 1g
carbs: 4g | fiber: 2g | sodium: 335mg

Crispy Artichokes with Lemon

Prep time: 10 minutes | Cook time: 15 minutes | Serves 2

Ingredients:

1 (15-ounce / 425-g) can artichoke hearts in water, drained
1 egg
1 tablespoon water
¼ cup whole wheat bread crumbs
¼ teaspoon salt
¼ teaspoon paprika
½ lemon

Directions:

1. Preheat the air fryer to 380ºF (193ºC).
2. In a medium shallow bowl, beat together the egg and water until frothy.
3. In a separate medium shallow bowl, mix together the bread crumbs, salt, and paprika.
4. Dip each artichoke heart into the egg mixture, then into the bread crumb mixture, coating the outside with the crumbs. Place the artichokes hearts in a single layer of the air fryer basket.
5. Fry the artichoke hearts for 15 minutes.
6. Remove the artichokes from the air fryer, and squeeze fresh lemon juice over the top before serving.

Per Serving

calories: 91 | fat: 2g | protein: 5g
carbs: 16g | fiber: 8g | sodium: 505mg

Ricotta Stuffed Bell Peppers

Prep time: 10 minutes | Cook time: 20 minutes | Serves 4

Ingredients:

2 red bell peppers
1 cup cooked brown rice
2 Roma tomatoes, diced
1 garlic clove, minced
¼ teaspoon salt
¼ teaspoon black pepper
4 ounces (113 g) ricotta
3 tablespoons fresh basil, chopped
3 tablespoons fresh oregano, chopped
¼ cup shredded Parmesan, for topping

Directions:

1. Preheat the air fryer to 360ºF (182ºC).
2. Cut the bell peppers in half and remove the seeds and stem.
3. In a medium bowl, combine the brown rice, tomatoes, garlic, salt, and pepper.
4. Distribute the rice filling evenly among the four bell pepper halves.
5. In a small bowl, combine the ricotta, basil, and oregano. Put the herbed cheese over the top of the rice mixture in each bell pepper.
6. Place the bell peppers into the air fryer and roast for 20 minutes.
7. Remove and serve with shredded Parmesan on top.

Per Serving

calories: 156 | fat: 6g | protein: 8g
carbs: 19g | fiber: 3g | sodium: 264mg

Vegetable Hummus Wraps

Prep time: 15 minutes | Cook time: 10 minutes | Serves 6

Ingredients:

1 large eggplant
1 large onion
½ cup extra-virgin olive oil
1 teaspoon salt
6 lavash wraps or large pita bread
1 cup hummus

Directions:

1. Preheat a grill, large grill pan, or lightly oiled large skillet on medium heat.
2. Slice the eggplant and onion into circles. Brush the vegetables with olive oil and sprinkle with salt.
3. Cook the vegetables on both sides, about 3 to 4 minutes each side.
4. To make the wrap, lay the lavash or pita flat. Spread about 2 tablespoons of hummus on the wrap.
5. Evenly divide the vegetables among the wraps, layering them along one side of the wrap. Gently fold over the side of the wrap with the vegetables, tucking them in and making a tight wrap.
6. Lay the wrap seam side-down and cut in half or thirds.
7. You can also wrap each sandwich with plastic wrap to help it hold its shape and eat it later.

Per Serving

calories: 362 | fat: 26g | protein: 15g
carbs: 28g | fiber: 11g | sodium: 1069mg

Lemon Green Beans with Red Onion

Prep time: 5 minutes | Cook time: 10 minutes | Serves 6

Ingredients:

1 pound (454 g) fresh green beans, trimmed
½ red onion, sliced
2 tablespoons olive oil
½ teaspoon salt
¼ teaspoon black pepper
1 tablespoon lemon juice
Lemon wedges, for serving

Directions:

1. Preheat the air fryer to 360ºF (182ºC). In a large bowl, toss the green beans, onion, olive oil, salt, pepper, and lemon juice until combined.
2. Pour the mixture into the air fryer and roast for 5 minutes. Stir well and roast for 5 minutes more.
3. Serve with lemon wedges.

Per Serving

calories: 67 | fat: 5g | protein: 1g
carbs: 6g | fiber: 2g | sodium: 199mg

Walnut Carrots with Honey Glaze

Prep time: 5 minutes | Cook time: 12 minutes | Serves 6

Ingredients:

1 pound (454 g) baby carrots
2 tablespoons olive oil
¼ cup raw honey
¼ teaspoon ground cinnamon
¼ cup black walnuts, chopped

Directions:

1. Preheat the air fryer to 360ºF (182ºC).
2. In a large bowl, toss the baby carrots with olive oil, honey, and cinnamon until well coated.
3. Pour into the air fryer and roast for 6 minutes. Shake the basket, sprinkle the walnuts on top, and roast for 6 minutes more.
4. Remove the carrots from the air fryer and serve.

Per Serving

calories: 146 | fat: 8g | protein: 1g
carbs: 20g | fiber: 3g | sodium: 60mg

Dill Beets

Prep time: 10 minutes | Cook time: 30 minutes | Serves 4

Ingredients:

4 beets, cleaned, peeled, and sliced
1 garlic clove, minced
2 tablespoons chopped fresh dill
¼ teaspoon salt
¼ teaspoon black pepper
3 tablespoons olive oil

Directions:

1. Preheat the air fryer to 380ºF (193ºC).
2. In a large bowl, mix together all of the ingredients so the beets are well coated with the oil.
3. Pour the beet mixture into the air fryer basket, and roast for 15 minutes before stirring, then continue roasting for 15 minutes more.

Per Serving

calories: 126 | fat: 10g | protein: 1g
carbs: 8g | fiber: 2g | sodium: 210mg

Orange-Honey Roasted Broccoli

Prep time: 5 minutes | Cook time: 12 minutes | Serves 6

Ingredients:

4 cups broccoli florets (approximately 1 large head)
2 tablespoons olive oil
½ teaspoon salt
½ cup orange juice
1 tablespoon raw honey
Orange wedges, for serving (optional)

Directions:

1. Preheat the air fryer to 360ºF (182ºC).
2. In a large bowl, combine the broccoli, olive oil, salt, orange juice, and honey. Toss the broccoli in the liquid until well coated.
3. Pour the broccoli mixture into the air fryer basket and cook for 6 minutes. Stir and cook for 6 minutes more.
4. Serve alone or with orange wedges for additional citrus flavor, if desired.

Per Serving

calories: 80 | fat: 5g | protein: 2g
carbs: 9g | fiber: 2g | sodium: 203mg

Parmesan Butternut Squash

Prep time: 15 minutes | Cook time: 20 minutes | Serves 4

Ingredients:

2½ cups butternut squash, cubed into 1-inch pieces (approximately 1 medium)
2 tablespoons olive oil
¼ teaspoon salt
¼ teaspoon garlic powder
¼ teaspoon black pepper
1 tablespoon fresh thyme
¼ cup grated Parmesan

Directions:

1. Preheat the air fryer to 360ºF (182ºC).
2. In a large bowl, combine the cubed squash with the olive oil, salt, garlic powder, pepper, and thyme until the squash is well coated.
3. Pour this mixture into the air fryer basket, and roast for 10 minutes. Stir and roast another 8 to 10 minutes more.
4. Remove the squash from the air fryer and toss with freshly grated Parmesan before serving.

Per Serving

calories: 127 | fat: 9g | protein: 3g
carbs: 11g | fiber: 2g | sodium: 262mg

Ratatouille

Prep time: 15 minutes | Cook time: 40 minutes | Serves 6

Ingredients:

2 russet potatoes, cubed
½ cup Roma tomatoes, cubed
1 eggplant, cubed
1 zucchini, cubed
1 red onion, chopped
1 red bell pepper, chopped
2 garlic cloves, minced
1 teaspoon dried mint
1 teaspoon dried parsley
1 teaspoon dried oregano
½ teaspoon salt
½ teaspoon black pepper
¼ teaspoon red pepper flakes
1/3 cup olive oil
1 (8-ounce / 227-g) can tomato paste
¼ cup vegetable broth
¼ cup water

Directions:

1. Preheat the air fryer to 320ºF (160ºC).
2. In a large bowl, combine the potatoes, tomatoes, eggplant, zucchini, onion, bell pepper, garlic, mint, parsley, oregano, salt, black pepper, and red pepper flakes.
3. In a small bowl, mix together the olive oil, tomato paste, broth, and water.
4. Pour the oil-and-tomato-paste mixture over the vegetables and toss until everything is coated.
5. Pour the coated vegetables into the air fryer basket in an even layer and roast for 20 minutes. After 20 minutes, stir well and spread out again. Roast for an additional 10 minutes, then repeat the process and cook for another 10 minutes.

Per Serving

calories: 280 | fat: 13g | protein: 6g
carbs: 40g | fiber: 7g | sodium: 264mg

Garlic Eggplant Slices

Prep time: 5 minutes | Cook time: 25 minutes | Serves 4

Ingredients:

1 egg
1 tablespoon water
½ cup whole wheat bread crumbs
1 teaspoon garlic powder
½ teaspoon dried oregano
½ teaspoon salt
½ teaspoon paprika
1 medium eggplant, sliced into ¼-inch-thick rounds
1 tablespoon olive oil

Directions:

1. Preheat the air fryer to 360ºF (182ºC).
2. In a medium shallow bowl, beat together the egg and water until frothy.
3. In a separate medium shallow bowl, mix together bread crumbs, garlic powder, oregano, salt, and paprika.
4. Dip each eggplant slice into the egg mixture, then into the bread crumb mixture, coating the outside with crumbs. Place the slices in a single layer in the bottom of the air fryer basket.
5. Drizzle the tops of the eggplant slices with the olive oil, then fry for 15 minutes. Turn each slice and cook for an additional 10 minutes.

Per Serving

calories: 137 | fat: 5g | protein: 5g
carbs: 19g | fiber: 5g | sodium: 409mg

Roasted Acorn Squash with Sage

Prep time: 10 minutes | Cook time: 35 minutes | Serves 6

Ingredients:

2 acorn squash, medium to large
2 tablespoons extra-virgin olive oil
1 teaspoon salt, plus more for seasoning
5 tablespoons unsalted butter
¼ cup chopped sage leaves
2 tablespoons fresh thyme leaves
½ teaspoon freshly ground black pepper

Directions:

1. Preheat the oven to 400ºF (205ºC).
2. Cut the acorn squash in half lengthwise. Scrape out the seeds with a spoon and cut it horizontally into ¾-inch-thick slices.
3. In a large bowl, drizzle the squash with the olive oil, sprinkle with salt, and toss together to coat.
4. Lay the acorn squash flat on a baking sheet.
5. Put the baking sheet in the oven and bake the squash for 20 minutes. Flip squash over with a spatula and bake for another 15 minutes.
6. Melt the butter in a medium saucepan over medium heat.
7. Add the sage and thyme to the melted butter and let them cook for 30 seconds.
8. Transfer the cooked squash slices to a plate. Spoon the butter/herb mixture over the squash. Season with salt and black pepper. Serve warm.

Per Serving

calories: 188 | fat: 15g | protein: 1g
carbs: 16g | fiber: 3g | sodium: 393mg

Spinach Cheese Pies

Prep time: 20 minutes | Cook time: 40 minutes | Serves 6 to 8

Ingredients:

2 tablespoons extra-virgin olive oil
1 large onion, chopped
2 cloves garlic, minced
3 (1-pound / 454-g) bags of baby spinach, washed
1 cup feta cheese
1 large egg, beaten
Puff pastry sheets

Directions:

1. Preheat the oven to 375ºF (190ºC).
2. In a large skillet over medium heat, cook the olive oil, onion, and garlic for 3 minutes.
3. Add the spinach to the skillet one bag at a time, letting it wilt in between each bag. Toss using tongs. Cook for 4 minutes. Once the spinach is cooked, drain any excess liquid from the pan.
4. In a large bowl, combine the feta cheese, egg, and cooked spinach.
5. Lay the puff pastry flat on a counter. Cut the pastry into 3-inch squares.
6. Place a tablespoon of the spinach mixture in the center of a puff-pastry square. Fold over one corner of the square to the diagonal corner, forming a triangle. Crimp the edges of the pie by pressing down with the tines of a fork to seal them together. Repeat until all squares are filled.
7. Place the pies on a parchment-lined baking sheet and bake for 25 to 30 minutes or until golden brown. Serve warm or at room temperature.

Per Serving

calories: 503 | fat: 32g | protein: 16g
carbs: 38g | fiber: 6g | sodium: 843mg

Carrot and Bean Stuffed Peppers

Prep time: 20 minutes | Cook time: 30 minutes | Serves 6

Ingredients:

6 large bell peppers, different colors
3 tablespoons extra-virgin olive oil
1 large onion, chopped
3 cloves garlic, minced
1 carrot, chopped

1 (16-ounce / 454-g) can garbanzo beans, rinsed and drained
3 cups cooked rice
1½ teaspoons salt
½ teaspoon freshly ground black pepper

Directions:

1. Preheat the oven to 350ºF (180ºC).
2. Make sure to choose peppers that can stand upright. Cut off the pepper cap and remove the seeds, reserving the cap for later. Stand the peppers in a baking dish.
3. In a large skillet over medium heat, cook the olive oil, onion, garlic, and carrots for 3 minutes.
4. Stir in the garbanzo beans. Cook for another 3 minutes.
5. Remove the pan from the heat and spoon the cooked ingredients to a large bowl.
6. Add the rice, salt, and pepper; toss to combine.
7. Stuff each pepper to the top and then put the pepper caps back on.
8. Cover the baking dish with aluminum foil and bake for 25 minutes.
9. Remove the foil and bake for another 5 minutes.
10. Serve warm.

Per Serving

calories: 301 | fat: 9g | protein: 8g | carbs: 50g | fiber: 8g | sodium: 597mg

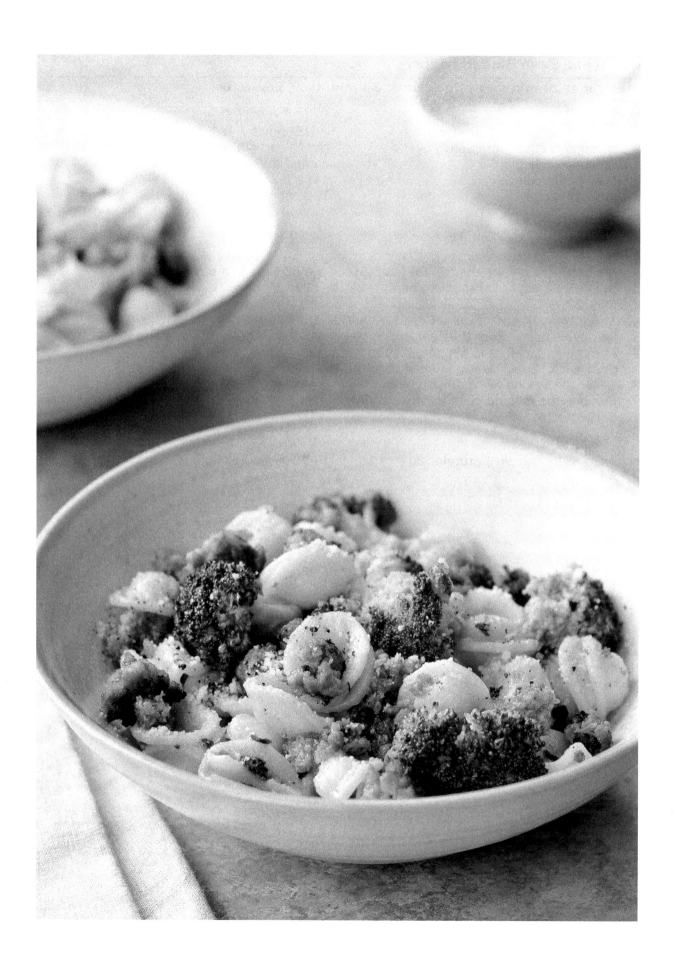

Chapter 4 Sides, Salads, and Soups

Beet Summer Salad

Prep time: 20 minutes | Cook time: 40 minutes | Serves 4 to 6

Ingredients:

6 medium to large fresh red or yellow beets
1/3 cup plus 1 tablespoon extra-virgin olive oil, divided
4 heads of Treviso radicchio
2 shallots, peeled and sliced
1/4 cup lemon juice
1/2 teaspoon salt
6 ounces (170 g) feta cheese, crumbled

Directions:

1. Preheat the oven to 400ºF (205ºC).
2. Cut off the stems and roots of the beets. Wash the beets thoroughly and dry them off with a paper towel.
3. Peel the beets using a vegetable peeler. Cut into ½-inch pieces and put them into a large bowl.
4. Add 1 tablespoon of olive oil to the bowl and toss to coat, then pour the beets out onto a baking sheet. Spread the beets so that they are evenly distributed.
5. Bake for 35 to 40 minutes until the beets are tender, turning once or twice with a spatula.
6. When the beets are done cooking, set them aside and let cool for 10 minutes.
7. While the beets are cooling, cut the radicchio into 1-inch pieces and place on a serving dish.
8. Once the beets have cooled, spoon them over the radicchio, then evenly distribute the shallots over the beets.
9. In a small bowl, whisk together the remaining 1/3 cup of olive oil, lemon juice, and salt. Drizzle the layered salad with dressing. Finish off the salad with feta cheese on top.

Per Serving

calories: 389 | fat: 31g | protein: 10g
carbs: 22g | fiber: 5g | sodium: 893mg

Balsamic Brussels Sprouts and Delicata Squash

Prep time: 10 minutes | Cook time: 30 minutes | Serves 2

Ingredients:

½ pound (227 g) Brussels sprouts, ends trimmed and outer leaves removed
1 medium delicata squash, halved lengthwise, seeded, and cut into 1-inch pieces
1 cup fresh cranberries
2 teaspoons olive oil
Salt and freshly ground black pepper, to taste
½ cup balsamic vinegar
2 tablespoons roasted pumpkin seeds
2 tablespoons fresh pomegranate arils (seeds)

Directions:

1. Preheat oven to 400ºF (205ºC) and set the rack to the middle position. Line a sheet pan with parchment paper.
2. Combine the Brussels sprouts, squash, and cranberries in a large bowl. Drizzle with olive oil, and season liberally with salt and pepper. Toss well to coat and arrange in a single layer on the sheet pan.
3. Roast for 30 minutes, turning vegetables halfway through, or until Brussels sprouts turn brown and crisp in spots and squash has golden-brown spots.
4. While vegetables are roasting, prepare the balsamic glaze by simmering the vinegar for 10 to 12 minutes, or until mixture has reduced to about ¼ cup and turns a syrupy consistency.
5. Remove the vegetables from the oven, drizzle with balsamic syrup, and sprinkle with pumpkin seeds and pomegranate arils before serving.

Per Serving

calories: 201 | fat: 7g | protein: 6g
carbs: 21g | fiber: 8g | sodium: 34mg

Lemon and Thyme Roasted Vegetables

Prep time: 20 minutes | Cook time: 50 minutes | Serves 2

Ingredients:

1 head garlic, cloves split apart, unpeeled
2 tablespoons olive oil, divided
2 medium carrots
¼ pound (113 g) asparagus
6 Brussels sprouts
2 cups cauliflower florets
½ pint cherry or grape tomatoes
½ fresh lemon, sliced
Salt and freshly ground black pepper, to taste
3 sprigs fresh thyme or ½ teaspoon dried thyme
Freshly squeezed lemon juice

Directions:

1. Preheat oven to 375ºF (190ºC) and set the rack to the middle position. Line a sheet pan with parchment paper or foil.
2. Place the garlic cloves in a small piece of foil and wrap lightly to enclose them, but don't seal the package. Drizzle with 1 teaspoon of olive oil. Place the foil packet on the sheet pan and roast for 30 minutes while you prepare the remaining vegetables.
3. While garlic is roasting, clean, peel, and trim vegetables: Cut carrots into strips, ½-inch wide and 3 to 4 inches long; snap tough ends off asparagus; trim tough ends off the Brussels sprouts and cut in half if they are large; trim cauliflower into 2-inch florets; keep tomatoes whole. The vegetables should be cut into pieces of similar size for even roasting.
4. Place all vegetables and the lemon slices into a large mixing bowl. Drizzle with the remaining 5 teaspoons of olive oil and season generously with salt and pepper.
5. Increase the oven temperature to 400ºF (205ºC).
6. Arrange the vegetables on the sheet pan in a single layer, leaving the packet of garlic cloves on the pan. Roast for 20 minutes, turning occasionally, until tender.
7. When the vegetables are tender, remove from the oven and sprinkle with thyme leaves. Let the garlic cloves sit until cool enough to handle, and then remove the skins. Leave them whole, or gently mash.
8. Toss garlic with the vegetables and an additional squeeze of fresh lemon juice.

Per Serving

calories: 256 | fat: 15g | protein: 7g
carbs: 31g | fiber: 9g | sodium: 168mg

Roasted Parmesan Rosemary Potatoes

Prep time: 10 minutes | Cook time: 55 minutes | Serves 2

Ingredients:

12 ounces (340 g) red potatoes (3 to 4 small potatoes)
1 tablespoon olive oil
½ teaspoon garlic powder
¼ teaspoon salt
1 tablespoon grated Parmesan cheese
1 teaspoon minced fresh rosemary (from 1 sprig)

Directions:

1. Preheat the oven to 425ºF (220ºC) and set the rack to the bottom position. Line a baking sheet with parchment paper. (Do not use foil, as the potatoes will stick.)
2. Scrub the potatoes and dry them well. Dice into 1-inch pieces.
3. In a mixing bowl, combine the potatoes, olive oil, garlic powder, and salt. Toss well to coat.
4. Lay the potatoes on the parchment paper and roast for 10 minutes. Flip the potatoes over and return to the oven for 10 more minutes.
5. Check the potatoes to make sure they are golden brown on the top and bottom. Toss them again, turn the heat down to 350ºF (180ºC), and roast for 30 minutes more.
6. When the potatoes are golden, crispy, and cooked through, sprinkle the Parmesan cheese over them and toss again. Return to the oven for 3 minutes to let the cheese melt a bit.
7. Remove from the oven and sprinkle with the fresh rosemary.

Per Serving

calories: 193 | fat: 8g | protein: 5g
carbs: 28g | fiber: 3g | sodium: 334mg

Spicy Wilted Greens

Prep time: 10 minutes | Cook time: 5 minutes | Serves 2

Ingredients:

1 tablespoon olive oil
2 garlic cloves, minced
3 cups sliced greens (kale, spinach, chard, beet greens, dandelion greens, or a combination)
Pinch salt
Pinch red pepper flakes (or more to taste)

Directions:

1. Heat the olive oil in a sauté pan over medium-high heat. Add garlic and sauté for 30 seconds, or just until it's fragrant.
2. Add the greens, salt, and pepper flakes and stir to combine. Let the greens wilt, but do not overcook. Remove the pan from the heat and serve.

Per Serving

calories: 91 | fat: 7g | protein: 1g
carbs: 7g | fiber: 3g | sodium: 111mg

Cauliflower Tabbouleh Salad

Prep time: 15 minutes | Cook time: 5 minutes | Serves 6

Ingredients:

6 tablespoons extra-virgin olive oil, divided
4 cups riced cauliflower
3 garlic cloves, finely minced
1½ teaspoons salt
½ teaspoon freshly ground black pepper
½ large cucumber, peeled, seeded, and chopped
½ cup chopped mint leaves
½ cup chopped Italian parsley
½ cup chopped pitted Kalamata olives
2 tablespoons minced red onion
Juice of 1 lemon (about 2 tablespoons)
2 cups baby arugula or spinach leaves
2 medium avocados, peeled, pitted, and diced
1 cup quartered cherry tomatoes

Directions:

1. In a large skillet, heat 2 tablespoons of olive oil over medium-high heat. Add the riced cauliflower, garlic, salt, and pepper and sauté until just tender but not mushy, 3 to 4 minutes. Remove from the heat and place in a large bowl.
2. Add the cucumber, mint, parsley, olives, red onion, lemon juice, and remaining 4 tablespoons olive oil and toss well. Place in the refrigerator, uncovered, and refrigerate for at least 30 minutes, or up to 2 hours.
3. Before serving, add the arugula, avocado, and tomatoes and toss to combine well. Season to taste with salt and pepper and serve cold or at room temperature.

Per Serving

calories: 235 | fat: 21g | protein: 4g
carbs: 12g | fiber: 6g | sodium: 623mg

Romano Broccolini

Prep time: 5 minutes | Cook time: 10 minutes | Serves 2

Ingredients:

1 bunch broccolini (about 5 ounces / 142 g)
1 tablespoon olive oil
½ teaspoon garlic powder
¼ teaspoon salt
2 tablespoons grated Romano cheese

Directions:

1. Preheat the oven to 400ºF (205ºC) and set the oven rack to the middle position. Line a sheet pan with parchment paper or foil.
2. Slice the tough ends off the broccolini and place in a medium bowl. Add the olive oil, garlic powder, and salt and toss to combine. Arrange broccolini on the lined sheet pan.
3. Roast for 7 minutes, flipping pieces over halfway through the roasting time.
4. Remove the pan from the oven and sprinkle the cheese over the broccolini. With a pair of tongs, carefully flip the pieces over to coat all sides. Return to the oven for another 2 to 3 minutes, or until the cheese melts and starts to turn golden.

Per Serving

calories: 114 | fat: 9g | protein: 4g
carbs: 5g | fiber: 2g | sodium: 400mg

Honey Roasted Rainbow Carrots

Prep time: 10 minutes | Cook time: 20 minutes | Serves 2

Ingredients:

½ pound (227 g) rainbow carrots (about 4)
2 tablespoons fresh orange juice
1 tablespoon honey
½ teaspoon coriander
Pinch salt

Directions:

1. Preheat oven to 400ºF (205ºC) and set the oven rack to the middle position.
2. Peel the carrots and cut them lengthwise into slices of even thickness. Place them in a large bowl.
3. In a small bowl, mix together the orange juice, honey, coriander, and salt.
4. Pour the orange juice mixture over the carrots and toss well to coat.
5. Spread carrots onto a baking dish in a single layer.
6. Roast for 15 to 20 minutes, or until fork-tender.

Per Serving

calories: 85 | fat: 0g | protein: 1g
carbs: 21g | fiber: 3g | sodium: 156mg

Garlicky Roasted Grape Tomatoes

Prep time: 10 minutes | Cook time: 45 minutes | Serves 2

Ingredients:

1 pint grape tomatoes
10 whole garlic cloves, skins removed
¼ cup olive oil
½ teaspoon salt
1 fresh rosemary sprig
1 fresh thyme sprig

Directions:

1. Preheat oven to 350ºF (180ºC).
2. Toss tomatoes, garlic cloves, oil, salt, and herb sprigs in a baking dish.
3. Roast tomatoes until they are soft and begin to caramelize, about 45 minutes.
4. Remove herbs before serving.

Per Serving

calories: 271 | fat: 26g | protein: 3g
carbs: 12g | fiber: 3g | sodium: 593mg

Homemade Vegetarian Chili

Prep time: 15 minutes | Cook time: 45 minutes | Serves 6 to 8

Ingredients:

2 tablespoons extra-virgin olive oil
2 carrots, peeled and chopped
½ large yellow onion, chopped
5 garlic cloves, minced
1 large zucchini, finely chopped
4 cups low-sodium vegetable broth
1 (14½-ounce / 411-g) can diced tomatoes
¼ cup tomato paste
2½ teaspoons chili powder
1 teaspoon sweet paprika
1 teaspoon ground cumin
½ teaspoon ground allspice
Salt and freshly ground black pepper, to taste
½ cup water
4 tablespoons gluten-free all-purpose flour
2 (15-ounce / 425-g) cans chickpeas, drained and rinsed
2 (15-ounce / 425-g) cans kidney beans, drained and rinsed
1 cup plain, unsweetened, full-fat Greek yogurt, for serving

Directions:

1. In a large pot, heat the olive oil over medium heat. Add the carrots, onion, and garlic and cook for about 4 minutes, tossing regularly, until softened. Add the zucchini and cook for about 4 minutes, until softened.
2. Add the broth, tomatoes and their juices, tomato paste, chili powder, paprika, cumin, and allspice. Season with salt and pepper. Bring to a boil.
3. Meanwhile, in a small bowl, pour in the water and the flour, stirring the flour in 1 tablespoon at a time, until mixed.
4. Mix chickpeas and kidney beans into the pot of chili and stir until completely combined. To thicken the chili, add the flour mixture 1 tablespoon at a time, stirring well with each addition. Lower the heat and simmer for 25 minutes, until thickened.
5. Serve with a dollop of full-fat, plain Greek yogurt.

Per Serving

calories: 430 | fat: 8g | protein: 22g
carbs: 67g | fiber: 17g | sodium: 354mg

Spinach and Zucchini Lasagna

Prep time: 15 minutes | Cook time: 1 hour | Serves 8

Ingredients:

½ cup extra-virgin olive oil, divided
4 to 5 medium zucchini squash
1 teaspoon salt
8 ounces (227 g) frozen spinach, thawed and well drained (about 1 cup)
2 cups whole-milk ricotta cheese
¼ cup chopped fresh basil or 2 teaspoons dried basil
1 teaspoon garlic powder
½ teaspoon freshly ground black pepper
2 cups shredded fresh whole-milk Mozzarella cheese
1¾ cups shredded Parmesan cheese
½ (24-ounce / 680-g) jar low-sugar marinara sauce (less than 5 grams sugar

Directions:

1. Preheat the oven to 425ºF (220ºC).
2. Line two baking sheets with parchment paper or aluminum foil and drizzle each with 2 tablespoons olive oil, spreading evenly.
3. Slice the zucchini lengthwise into ¼-inch-thick long slices and place on the prepared baking sheet in a single layer. Sprinkle with ½ teaspoon salt per sheet. Bake until softened, but not mushy, 15 to 18 minutes. Remove from the oven and allow to cool slightly before assembling the lasagna.
4. Reduce the oven temperature to 375ºF (190ºC).
5. While the zucchini cooks, prep the filling. In a large bowl, combine the spinach, ricotta, basil, garlic powder, and pepper. In a small bowl, mix together the Mozzarella and Parmesan cheeses. In a medium bowl, combine the marinara sauce and remaining ¼ cup olive oil and stir to fully incorporate the oil into sauce.
6. To assemble the lasagna, spoon a third of the marinara sauce mixture into the bottom of a 9-by-13-inch glass baking dish and spread evenly. Place 1 layer of softened zucchini slices to fully cover the sauce, then add a third of the ricotta-spinach mixture and spread evenly on top of the zucchini. Sprinkle a third of the Mozzarella-Parmesan mixture on top of the ricotta. Repeat with 2 more cycles of these layers: marinara, zucchini, ricotta-spinach, then cheese blend.
7. Bake until the cheese is bubbly and melted, 30 to 35 minutes. Turn the broiler to low and broil until the top is golden brown, about 5 minutes. Remove from the oven and allow to cool slightly before slicing.

Per Serving

calories: 521 | fat: 41g | protein: 25g
carbs: 13g | fiber: 3g | sodium: 712mg

Tomato and Lentil Salad with Feta

Prep time: 10 minutes | Cook time: 30 minutes | Serves 4

Ingredients:

3 cups water
1 cup brown or green lentils, picked over and rinsed
1½ teaspoons salt, divided
2 large ripe tomatoes
2 Persian cucumbers
⅓ cup lemon juice
½ cup extra-virgin olive oil
1 cup crumbled feta cheese

Directions:

1. In a large pot over medium heat, bring the water, lentils, and 1 teaspoon of salt to a simmer, then reduce heat to low. Cover the pot and continue to cook, stirring occasionally, for 30 minutes. (The lentils should be cooked so that they no longer have a crunch, but still hold their form. You should be able to smooth the lentil between your two fingers when pinched.)
2. Once the lentils are done cooking, strain them to remove any excess water and put them into a large bowl. Let cool.
3. Dice the tomatoes and cucumbers, then add them to the lentils.
4. In a small bowl, whisk together the lemon juice, olive oil, and remaining ½ teaspoon salt.
5. Pour the dressing over the lentils and vegetables. Add the feta cheese to the bowl, and gently toss all of the ingredients together.

Per Serving

calories: 521 | fat: 36g | protein: 18g
carbs: 35g | fiber: 15g | sodium: 1304mg

Pistachio Citrus Asparagus

Prep time: 10 minutes | Cook time: 15 minutes | Serves 4

Ingredients:

5 tablespoons extra-virgin olive oil, divided
Zest and juice of 2 clementines or 1 orange (about ¼ cup juice and 1 tablespoon zest)
Zest and juice of 1 lemon
1 tablespoon red wine vinegar
1 teaspoon salt, divided
¼ teaspoon freshly ground black pepper
½ cup shelled pistachios
1 pound (454 g) fresh asparagus
1 tablespoon water

Directions:

1. In a small bowl, whisk together 4 tablespoons olive oil, the clementine and lemon juices and zests, vinegar, ½ teaspoon salt, and pepper. Set aside.
2. In a medium dry skillet, toast the pistachios over medium-high heat until lightly browned, 2 to 3 minutes, being careful not to let them burn. Transfer to a cutting board and coarsely chop. Set aside.
3. Trim the rough ends off the asparagus, usually the last 1 to 2 inches of each spear. In a skillet, heat the remaining 1 tablespoon olive oil over medium-high heat. Add the asparagus and sauté for 2 to 3 minutes. Sprinkle with the remaining ½ teaspoon salt and add the water. Reduce the heat to medium-low, cover, and cook until tender, another 2 to 4 minutes, depending on the thickness of the spears.
4. Transfer the cooked asparagus to a serving dish. Add the pistachios to the dressing and whisk to combine. Pour the dressing over the warm asparagus and toss to coat.

Per Serving

calories: 284 | fat: 24g | protein: 6g
carbs: 11g | fiber: 4g | sodium: 594mg

Pasta Bean Soup

Prep time: 5 minutes | Cook time: 25 minutes | Serves 6

Ingredients:

2 tablespoons extra-virgin olive oil
½ cup chopped onion (about ¼ onion)
3 garlic cloves, minced (about 1½ teaspoons)
1 tablespoon minced fresh rosemary or 1 teaspoon dried rosemary
¼ teaspoon crushed red pepper
4 cups low-sodium or no-salt-added vegetable broth
2 (15½-ounce / 439-g) cans cannellini, great northern, or light kidney beans, undrained
1 (28-ounce / 794-g) can low-sodium or no-salt-added crushed tomatoes
2 tablespoons tomato paste
8 ounces (227 g) uncooked short pasta, such as ditalini, tubetti, or elbows
6 tablespoons grated Parmesan cheese (about 1½ ounces / 43 g)

Directions:

1. In a large stockpot over medium heat, heat the oil. Add the onion and cook for 4 minutes, stirring frequently. Add the garlic, rosemary, and crushed red pepper. Cook for 1 minute, stirring frequently. Add the broth, canned beans with their liquid, tomatoes, and tomato paste. Simmer for 5 minutes.
2. To thicken the soup, carefully transfer 2 cups to a blender. Purée, then stir it back into the pot.
3. Bring the soup to a boil over high heat. Mix in the pasta, and lower the heat to a simmer. Cook the pasta for the amount of time recommended on the box, stirring every few minutes to prevent the pasta from sticking to the pot. Taste the pasta to make sure it is cooked through (it could take a few more minutes than the recommended cooking time, since it's cooking with other ingredients).
4. Ladle the soup into bowls, top each with 1 tablespoon of grated cheese, and serve.

Per Serving

calories: 583 | fat: 6g | protein: 32g
carbs: 103g | fiber: 29g | sodium: 234mg

Quinoa and Garbanzo Salad

Prep time: 10 minutes | Cook time: 30 minutes | Serves 8

Ingredients:

4 cups water
2 cups red or yellow quinoa
2 teaspoons salt, divided
1 cup thinly sliced onions (red or white)
1 (16-ounce / 454-g)

can garbanzo beans, rinsed and drained
1/3 cup extra-virgin olive oil
¼ cup lemon juice
1 teaspoon freshly ground black pepper

Directions:

1. In a 3-quart pot over medium heat, bring the water to a boil.
2. Add the quinoa and 1 teaspoon of salt to the pot. Stir, cover, and let cook over low heat for 15 to 20 minutes.
3. Turn off the heat, fluff the quinoa with a fork, cover again, and let stand for 5 to 10 more minutes.
4. Put the cooked quinoa, onions, and garbanzo beans in a large bowl.
5. In a separate small bowl, whisk together the olive oil, lemon juice, remaining 1 teaspoon of salt, and black pepper.
6. Add the dressing to the quinoa mixture and gently toss everything together. Serve warm or cold.

Per Serving

calories: 318 | fat: 6g | protein: 9g
carbs: 43g | fiber: 13g | sodium: 585mg

Winter Salad with Red Wine Vinaigrette

Prep time: 10 minutes | Cook time: 0 minutes | Serves 4

Ingredients:

1 small green apple, thinly sliced
6 stalks kale, stems removed and greens roughly chopped
½ cup crumbled feta cheese
½ cup dried currants
½ cup chopped pitted Kalamata olives
½ cup thinly sliced radicchio

2 scallions, both green and white parts, thinly sliced
¼ cup peeled, julienned carrots
2 celery stalks, thinly sliced
¼ cup Red Wine Vinaigrette
Salt and freshly ground black pepper, to taste (optional)

Directions:

1. In a large bowl, combine the apple, kale, feta, currants, olives, radicchio, scallions, carrots, and celery and mix well. Drizzle with the vinaigrette. Season with salt and pepper (if using), then serve.

Per Serving

calories: 253 | fat: 15g | protein: 6g
carbs: 29g | fiber: 4g | sodium: 480mg

Garlic Broccoli with Artichoke Hearts

Prep time: 5 minutes | Cook time: 10 minutes | Serves 4

Ingredients:

2 pounds (907 g) fresh broccoli rabe
½ cup extra-virgin olive oil, divided
3 garlic cloves, finely minced
1 teaspoon salt
1 teaspoon red pepper flakes

1 (13¾-ounce / 390-g) can artichoke hearts, drained and quartered
1 tablespoon water
2 tablespoons red wine vinegar
Freshly ground black pepper, to taste

Directions:

1. Trim away any thick lower stems and yellow leaves from the broccoli rabe and discard. Cut into individual florets with a couple inches of thin stem attached.
2. In a large skillet, heat ¼ cup olive oil over medium-high heat. Add the trimmed broccoli, garlic, salt, and red pepper flakes and sauté for 5 minutes, until the broccoli begins to soften. Add the artichoke hearts and sauté for another 2 minutes.
3. Add the water and reduce the heat to low. Cover and simmer until the broccoli stems are tender, 3 to 5 minutes.
4. In a small bowl, whisk together remaining ¼ cup olive oil and the vinegar. Drizzle over the broccoli and artichokes. Season with ground black pepper, if desired.

Per Serving

calories: 358 | fat: 35g | protein: 11g
carbs: 18g | fiber: 10g | sodium: 918mg

Roasted Lemon Tahini Cauliflower

Prep time: 10 minutes | Cook time: 20 minutes | Serves 2

Ingredients:

½ large head cauliflower, stemmed and broken into florets (about 3 cups)
1 tablespoon olive oil
2 tablespoons tahini

2 tablespoons freshly squeezed lemon juice
1 teaspoon harissa paste
Pinch salt

Directions:

1. Preheat the oven to 400ºF (205ºC) and set the rack to the lowest position. Line a sheet pan with parchment paper or foil.
2. Toss the cauliflower florets with the olive oil in a large bowl and transfer to the sheet pan. Reserve the bowl to make the tahini sauce.
3. Roast the cauliflower for 15 minutes, turning it once or twice, until it starts to turn golden.
4. In the same bowl, combine the tahini, lemon juice, harissa, and salt.
5. When the cauliflower is tender, remove it from the oven and toss it with the tahini sauce. Return to the sheet pan and roast for 5 minutes more.

Per Serving

calories: 205 | fat: 15g | protein: 7g
carbs: 15g | fiber: 7g | sodium: 161mg

Avocado and Hearts of Palm Salad

Prep time: 10 minutes | Cook time: 0 minutes | Serves 4

Ingredients:

2 (14-ounce / 397-g) cans hearts of palm, drained and cut into ½-inch-thick slices
1 avocado, cut into ½-inch pieces
1 cup halved yellow cherry tomatoes
½ small shallot, thinly sliced

¼ cup coarsely chopped flat-leaf parsley
2 tablespoons low-fat mayonnaise
2 tablespoons extra-virgin olive oil
¼ teaspoon salt
⅛ teaspoon freshly ground black pepper

Directions:

1. In a large bowl, toss the hearts of palm, avocado, tomatoes, shallot, and parsley.
2. In a small bowl, whisk the mayonnaise, olive oil, salt, and pepper, then mix into the large bowl.

Per Serving

calories: 192 | fat: 15g | protein: 5g
carbs: 14g | fiber: 7g | sodium: 841mg

Herb-Roasted Vegetables

Prep time: 15 minutes | Cook time: 45 minutes | Serves 6

Ingredients:

Nonstick cooking spray
2 eggplants, peeled and sliced ⅛ inch thick
1 zucchini, sliced ¼ inch thick
1 yellow summer squash, sliced ¼ inch thick
2 Roma tomatoes, sliced ⅛ inch thick
¼ cup, plus 2

tablespoons extra-virgin olive oil, divided
1 tablespoon garlic powder
¼ teaspoon dried oregano
¼ teaspoon dried basil
¼ teaspoon salt
Freshly ground black pepper, to taste

Directions:

1. Preheat the oven to 400ºF (205ºC).
2. Spray a 9-by-13-inch baking dish with cooking spray. In the dish, toss the eggplant, zucchini, squash, and tomatoes with 2 tablespoons oil, garlic powder, oregano, basil, salt, and pepper.
3. Standing the vegetables up (like little soldiers), alternate layers of eggplant, zucchini, squash, and Roma tomato.
4. Drizzle the top with the remaining ¼ cup of olive oil.
5. Bake, uncovered, for 40 to 45 minutes, or until vegetables are golden brown.

Per Serving

calories: 186 | fat: 14g | protein: 3g
carbs: 15g | fiber: 5g | sodium: 110mg

Tahini Barley Salad

Prep time: 20 minutes | Cook time: 8 minutes | Serves 4 to 6

Ingredients:

1½ cups pearl barley
5 tablespoons extra-virgin olive oil, divided
1½ teaspoons table salt, for cooking barley
¼ cup tahini
1 teaspoon grated lemon zest plus ¼ cup juice (2 lemons)
1 tablespoon sumac, divided
1 garlic clove, minced
¾ teaspoon table

salt
1 English cucumber, cut into ½-inch pieces
1 carrot, peeled and shredded
1 red bell pepper, stemmed, seeded, and chopped
4 scallions, thinly sliced
2 tablespoons finely chopped jarred hot cherry peppers
¼ cup coarsely chopped fresh mint

Directions:

1. Combine 6 cups water, barley, 1 tablespoon oil, and 1½ teaspoons salt in Instant Pot. Lock lid in place and close pressure release valve. Select high pressure cook function and cook for 8 minutes. Turn off Instant Pot and let pressure release naturally for 15 minutes. Quick-release any remaining pressure, then carefully remove lid, allowing steam to escape away from you. Drain barley, spread onto rimmed baking sheet, and let cool completely, about 15 minutes.
2. Meanwhile, whisk remaining ¼ cup oil, tahini, 2 tablespoons water, lemon zest and juice, 1 teaspoon sumac, garlic, and ¾ teaspoon salt in large bowl until combined; let sit for 15 minutes.
3. Measure out and reserve ½ cup dressing for serving. Add barley, cucumber, carrot, bell pepper, scallions, and cherry peppers to bowl with dressing and gently toss to combine. Season with salt and pepper to taste. Transfer salad to serving dish and sprinkle with mint and remaining 2 teaspoons sumac. Serve, passing reserved dressing separately.

Per Serving

calories: 370 | fat: 18g | protein: 8g
carbs: 47g | fiber: 10g | sodium: 510mg

French Green Lentils with Chard

Prep time: 15 minutes | Cook time: 20 minutes | Serves 6

Ingredients:

2 tablespoons extra-virgin olive oil, plus extra for drizzling
12 ounces (340 g) Swiss chard, stems chopped fine, leaves sliced into ½-inch-wide strips
1 onion, chopped fine
½ teaspoon table salt
2 garlic cloves, minced
1 teaspoon minced fresh thyme or ¼

teaspoon dried
2½ cups water
1 cup French green lentils, picked over and rinsed
3 tablespoons whole-grain mustard
½ teaspoon grated lemon zest plus 1 teaspoon juice
3 tablespoons sliced almonds, toasted
2 tablespoons chopped fresh parsley

Directions:

1. Using highest sauté function, heat oil in Instant Pot until shimmering. Add chard stems, onion, and salt and cook until vegetables are softened, about 5 minutes. Stir in garlic and thyme and cook until fragrant, about 30 seconds. Stir in water and lentils.
2. Lock lid in place and close pressure release valve. Select high pressure cook function and cook for 11 minutes. Turn off Instant Pot and let pressure release naturally for 15 minutes. Quick-release any remaining pressure, then carefully remove lid, allowing steam to escape away from you.
3. Stir chard leaves into lentils, 1 handful at a time, and let cook in residual heat until wilted, about 5 minutes. Stir in mustard and lemon zest and juice. Season with salt and pepper to taste. Transfer to serving dish, drizzle with extra oil, and sprinkle with almonds and parsley. Serve.

Per Serving

calories: 190 | fat: 8g | protein: 9g
carbs: 23g | fiber: 6g | sodium: 470mg

Arugula, Watermelon, and Feta Salad

Prep time: 10 minutes | Cook time: 0 minutes | Serves 2

Ingredients:

3 cups packed arugula
2½ cups watermelon, cut into bite-size cubes

2 ounces (57 g) feta cheese, crumbled
2 tablespoons balsamic glaze

Directions:

1. Divide the arugula between two plates.
2. Divide the watermelon cubes between the beds of arugula.
3. Sprinkle 1 ounce (28 g) of the feta over each salad.
4. Drizzle about 1 tablespoon of the glaze (or more if desired) over each salad.

Per Serving

calories: 159 | fat: 7g | protein: 6g
carbs: 21g | fiber: 1g | sodium: 327mg

Lentil Soup

Prep time: 25 minutes | Cook time: 1 hour 20 minutes | Serves 6 to 8

Ingredients:

10 cups water
2 cups brown lentils, picked over and rinsed
2 teaspoons salt, divided
¼ cup long-grain rice, rinsed
3 tablespoons extra-

virgin olive oil
1 large onion, chopped
2 medium potatoes, peeled
1 teaspoon ground cumin
½ teaspoon freshly ground black pepper

Directions:

1. In a large pot over medium heat, bring the water, lentils, and 1 teaspoon of salt to a simmer and continue to cook, stirring occasionally, for 30 minutes.
2. At the 30-minute mark, add the rice to the lentils. Cover and continue to simmer, stirring occasionally, for another 30 minutes.
3. Remove the pot from the heat and, using a handheld immersion blender, blend the lentils and rice for 1 to 2 minutes until smooth.
4. Return the pot to the stove over low heat.

5. In a small skillet over medium heat, cook the olive oil and onions for 5 minutes until the onions are golden brown. Add the onions to the soup.
6. Cut the potatoes into ¼-inch pieces and add them to the soup.
7. Add remaining 1 teaspoon of salt, cumin, and black pepper to the soup. Stir and continue to cook for 10 to 15 minutes, or until potatoes are thoroughly cooked. Serve warm.

Per Serving

calories: 348 | fat: 9g | protein: 18g
carbs: 53g | fiber: 20g | sodium: 795mg

Lemon Chicken Orzo Soup

Prep time: 10 minutes | Cook time: 20 minutes | Serves 8

Ingredients:

1 tablespoon extra-virgin olive oil
1 cup chopped onion
½ cup chopped carrots
½ cup chopped celery
3 garlic cloves, minced
9 cups low-sodium chicken broth
2 cups shredded

cooked chicken breast
½ cup freshly squeezed lemon juice
Zest of 1 lemon, grated
1 to 2 teaspoons dried oregano
8 ounces (227 g) cooked orzo pasta

Directions:

1. In a large pot, heat the oil over medium heat and add the onion, carrots, celery, and garlic and cook for about 5 minutes, until the onions are translucent. Add the broth and bring to a boil.
2. Reduce to a simmer, cover, and cook for 10 more minutes, until the flavors meld. Then add the shredded chicken, lemon juice and zest, and oregano.
3. Plate the orzo in serving bowls first, then add the chicken soup.

Per Serving

calories: 215 | fat: 5g | protein: 16g
carbs: 27g | fiber: 2g | sodium: 114mg

Tomato Basil Soup

Prep time: 10 minutes | Cook time: 10 minutes | Serves 2

Ingredients:

¼ cup extra-virgin olive oil
2 garlic cloves, minced
1 (14½-ounce / 411-g) can plum
tomatoes, whole or diced
1 cup vegetable broth
¼ cup chopped fresh basil

Directions:

1. In a medium pot, heat the oil over medium heat, then add the garlic and cook for 2 minutes, until fragrant.
2. Meanwhile, in a bowl using an immersion blender or in a blender, purée the tomatoes and their juices.
3. Add the puréed tomatoes and broth to the pot and mix well. Simmer for 10 to 15 minutes and serve, garnished with basil.

Per Serving

calories: 307 | fat: 27g | protein: 3g
carbs: 11g | fiber: 4g | sodium: 661mg

White Bean Soup with Kale

Prep time: 25 minutes | Cook time: 30 minutes | Serves 4

Ingredients:

1 to 2 tablespoons extra-virgin olive oil
1 large shallot, minced
1 large purple carrot, chopped
1 celery stalk, chopped
1 teaspoon garlic powder
3 cups low-sodium vegetable broth
1 (15-ounce / 425-g) can cannellini beans
1 cup chopped baby
kale
1 teaspoon salt (optional)
½ teaspoon freshly ground black pepper (optional)
1 lemon, juiced and zested
1½ tablespoons chopped fresh thyme (optional)
3 tablespoons chopped fresh oregano (optional)

Directions:

1. In a large, deep pot, heat the oil. Add the shallot, carrot, celery, and garlic powder and sauté on medium-low heat for 3 to 5 minutes, until the vegetables are golden.
2. Add the vegetable broth and beans and bring to a simmer. Cook for 15 minutes.
3. Add in the kale, salt (if using), and pepper (if using). Cook for another 5 to 10 minutes, until the kale is soft. Right before serving, stir in the lemon juice and zest, thyme (if using), and oregano (if using).

Per Serving

calories: 165 | fat: 4g | protein: 7g
carbs: 26g | fiber: 7g | sodium: 135mg

Hearty Mushroom Stew

Prep time: 10 minutes | Cook time: 40 minutes | Serves 6

Ingredients:

2 tablespoons extra-virgin olive oil
5 ounces (142 g) mushrooms, sliced
½ cup diced carrots
½ cup diced yellow onion
½ cup diced celery
2½ cups low-sodium vegetable broth
1 cup diced tomatoes
1 teaspoon garlic powder
1 bay leaf
1 russet potato, peeled and finely diced
1 cup cooked chickpeas
½ cup crumbled feta, for serving

Directions:

1. In a large sauté pan or skillet, heat the oil over medium heat. Add the mushrooms and cook for 5 minutes, until they reduce in size and soften.
2. Add the carrots, onion, and celery to the pan and cook for 10 minutes, or until the onions are golden. Pour in the vegetable broth, tomatoes, garlic powder, and bay leaf and bring to a simmer. Add the potato.
3. Mix well and cover. Cook for 20 minutes or until the potato is fork-tender.
4. Add in the chickpeas, stir, and the remove the bay leaf. Season with salt and pepper. Serve, topped with feta, and enjoy!

Per Serving

calories: 162 | fat: 8g | protein: 6g
carbs: 19g | fiber: 4g | sodium: 218mg

Tuna Salad

Prep time: 10 minutes | Cook time: 0 minutes | Serves 4

Ingredients:

4 cups spring mix greens

1 (15-ounce / 425-g) can cannellini beans, drained

2 (5-ounce / 142-g) cans water-packed, white albacore tuna, drained

⅔ cup crumbled feta cheese

½ cup thinly sliced sun-dried tomatoes

¼ cup sliced pitted Kalamata olives

¼ cup thinly sliced scallions, both green and white parts

3 tablespoons extra-virgin olive oil

½ teaspoon dried cilantro

2 or 3 leaves thinly chopped fresh sweet basil

1 lime, zested and juiced

Kosher salt and freshly ground black pepper, to taste

Directions:

1. In a large bowl, combine greens, beans, tuna, feta, tomatoes, olives, scallions, olive oil, cilantro, basil, and lime juice and zest. Season with salt and pepper, mix, and enjoy!

Per Serving (1 cup)

calories: 355 | fat: 19g | protein: 22g
carbs: 25g | fiber: 8g | sodium: 744mg

Mediterranean Bruschetta Hummus Platter

Prep time: 15 minutes | Cook time: 0 minutes | Serves 6

Ingredients:

½ cup finely diced fresh tomato

⅓ cup finely diced seedless English cucumber

1 teaspoon extra-virgin olive oil

1 (10-ounce / 283-g) container plain hummus

2 tablespoons balsamic glaze

2 tablespoons crumbled feta cheese

1 tablespoon fresh chopped parsley or basil

¼ cup Herbed Olive Oil

4 warmed pitas, cut into wedges, for serving

Carrot sticks, for serving

Celery sticks, for serving

Sliced bell peppers, for serving

Broccoli, for serving

Purple cauliflower, for serving

Directions:

1. In a small bowl, mix the tomato and cucumber and toss with the olive oil. Pile the cucumber mixture over a fresh container of hummus. Drizzle the hummus and vegetables with the balsamic glaze. Top with crumbled feta and fresh parsley.
2. Put the hummus on a large cutting board. Pour the Herbed Olive Oil in a small bowl and put it on the cutting board. Surround the bowls with the pita wedges and cut carrot sticks, celery sticks, sliced bell peppers, broccoli, and cauliflower.

Per Serving

calories: 345 | fat: 19g | protein: 9g
carbs: 32g | fiber: 3g | sodium: 473mg

Arugula and Walnut Salad

Prep time: 10 minutes | Cook time: 0 minutes | Serves 4

Ingredients:

4 tablespoons extra-virgin olive oil

Zest and juice of 2 clementines or 1 orange (2 to 3 tablespoons)

1 tablespoon red wine vinegar

½ teaspoon salt

¼ teaspoon freshly ground black pepper

8 cups baby arugula

1 cup coarsely chopped walnuts

1 cup crumbled goat cheese

½ cup pomegranate seeds

Directions:

1. In a small bowl, whisk together the olive oil, zest and juice, vinegar, salt, and pepper and set aside.
2. To assemble the salad for serving, in a large bowl, combine the arugula, walnuts, goat cheese, and pomegranate seeds. Drizzle with the dressing and toss to coat.

Per Serving

calories: 444 | fat: 40g | protein: 10g
carbs: 11g | fiber: 3g | sodium: 412mg

Kale Salad with Anchovy Dressing

Prep time: 15 minutes | Cook time: 0 minutes | Serves 4

Ingredients:

1 large bunch lacinato or dinosaur kale
¼ cup toasted pine nuts
1 cup shaved or coarsely shredded fresh Parmesan cheese
¼ cup extra-virgin

olive oil
8 anchovy fillets, roughly chopped
2 to 3 tablespoons freshly squeezed lemon juice (from 1 large lemon)
2 teaspoons red pepper flakes (optional)

Directions:

1. Remove the rough center stems from the kale leaves and roughly tear each leaf into about 4-by-1-inch strips. Place the torn kale in a large bowl and add the pine nuts and cheese.
2. In a small bowl, whisk together the olive oil, anchovies, lemon juice, and red pepper flakes (if using). Drizzle over the salad and toss to coat well. Let sit at room temperature 30 minutes before serving, tossing again just prior to serving.

Per Serving

calories: 337 | fat: 25g | protein: 16g
carbs: 12g | fiber: 2g | sodium: 603mg

Authentic Greek Salad

Prep time: 10 minutes | Cook time: 0 minutes | Serves 4

Ingredients:

2 large English cucumbers
4 Roma tomatoes, quartered
1 green bell pepper, cut into 1- to 1½-inch chunks
¼ small red onion, thinly sliced
4 ounces (113 g) pitted Kalamata olives
¼ cup extra-virgin olive oil
2 tablespoons freshly

squeezed lemon juice
1 tablespoon red wine vinegar
1 tablespoon chopped fresh oregano or 1 teaspoon dried oregano
¼ teaspoon freshly ground black pepper
4 ounces (113 g) crumbled traditional feta cheese

Directions:

1. Cut the cucumbers in half lengthwise and then into ½-inch-thick half-moons. Place in a large bowl.
2. Add the quartered tomatoes, bell pepper, red onion, and olives.
3. In a small bowl, whisk together the olive oil, lemon juice, vinegar, oregano, and pepper. Drizzle over the vegetables and toss to coat.
4. Divide between salad plates and top each with 1 ounce (28 g) of feta.

Per Serving

calories: 278 | fat: 22g | protein: 8g
carbs: 12g | fiber: 4g | sodium: 572mg

Greek Chicken Artichoke Soup

Prep time: 10 minutes | Cook time: 15 minutes | Serves 4

Ingredients:

4 cups chicken stock
2 cups riced cauliflower, divided
2 large egg yolks
¼ cup freshly squeezed lemon juice (about 2 lemons)
¾ cup extra-virgin olive oil, divided

8 ounces (227 g) cooked chicken, coarsely chopped
1 (13¾-ounce / 390-g) can artichoke hearts, drained and quartered
¼ cup chopped fresh dill

Directions:

1. In a large saucepan, bring the stock to a low boil. Reduce the heat to low and simmer, covered.
2. Transfer 1 cup of the hot stock to a blender or food processor. Add ½ cup raw riced cauliflower, the egg yolks, and lemon juice and purée. While the processor or blender is running, stream in ½ cup olive oil and blend until smooth.
3. Whisking constantly, pour the purée into the simmering stock until well blended together and smooth. Add the chicken and artichokes and simmer until thickened slightly, 8 to 10 minutes. Stir in the dill and remaining 1½ cups riced cauliflower. Serve warm, drizzled with the remaining ¼ cup olive oil.

Per Serving

calories: 566 | fat: 46g | protein: 24g
carbs: 14g | fiber: 7g | sodium: 754mg

Moroccan Lamb Lentil Soup

Prep time: 15 minutes | Cook time: 28 minutes | Serves 6 to 8

Ingredients:

1 pound (454 g) lamb shoulder chops (blade or round bone), 1 to 1½ inches thick, trimmed and halved
¾ teaspoon table salt, divided
⅛ teaspoon pepper
1 tablespoon extra-virgin olive oil
1 onion, chopped fine
¼ cup harissa, plus extra for serving
1 tablespoon all-purpose flour
8 cups chicken broth
1 cup French green lentils, picked over and rinsed
1 (15-ounce / 425-g) can chickpeas, rinsed
2 tomatoes, cored and cut into ¼-inch pieces
½ cup chopped fresh cilantro

Directions:

1. Pat lamb dry with paper towels and sprinkle with ¼ teaspoon salt and pepper. Using highest sauté function, heat oil in Instant Pot for 5 minutes (or until just smoking). Place lamb in pot and cook until well browned on first side, about 4 minutes; transfer to plate.
2. Add onion and remaining ½ teaspoon salt to fat left in pot and cook, using highest sauté function, until softened, about 5 minutes. Stir in harissa and flour and cook until fragrant, about 30 seconds. Slowly whisk in broth, scraping up any browned bits and smoothing out any lumps. Stir in lentils, then nestle lamb into multicooker and add any accumulated juices.
3. Lock lid in place and close pressure release valve. Select high pressure cook function and cook for 10 minutes. Turn off Instant Pot and quick-release pressure. Carefully remove lid, allowing steam to escape away from you.
4. Transfer lamb to cutting board, let cool slightly, then shred into bite-size pieces using 2 forks; discard excess fat and bones. Stir lamb and chickpeas into soup and let sit until heated through, about 3 minutes. Season with salt and pepper to taste. Top individual portions with tomatoes and sprinkle with cilantro. Serve, passing extra harissa separately.

Per Serving

calories: 300 | fat: 13g | protein: 22g
carbs: 24g | fiber: 6g | sodium: 940mg

Paella Soup

Prep time: 5 minutes | Cook time: 25 minutes | Serves 6

Ingredients:

1 cup frozen green peas
2 tablespoons extra-virgin olive oil
1 cup chopped onion (about ½ medium onion)
1½ cups coarsely chopped red bell pepper (about 1 large pepper)
1½ cups coarsely chopped green bell pepper (about 1 large pepper)
2 garlic cloves, chopped (about 1 teaspoon)
1 teaspoon ground turmeric
1 teaspoon dried thyme
2 teaspoons smoked paprika
2½ cups uncooked instant brown rice
2 cups low-sodium or no-salt-added chicken broth
2½ cups water
1 (28-ounce / 794-g) can low-sodium or no-salt-added crushed tomatoes
1 pound (454 g) fresh raw medium shrimp (or frozen raw shrimp completely thawed), shells and tails removed

Directions:

1. Put the frozen peas on the counter to partially thaw as the soup is being prepared.
2. In a large stockpot over medium-high heat, heat the oil. Add the onion, red and green bell peppers, and garlic. Cook for 8 minutes, stirring occasionally. Add the turmeric, thyme, and smoked paprika, and cook for 2 minutes more, stirring often. Stir in the rice, broth, and water. Bring to a boil over high heat. Cover, reduce the heat to medium-low, and cook for 10 minutes.
3. Stir the peas, tomatoes, and shrimp into the soup. Cook for 4 to 6 minutes, until the shrimp is cooked, turning from gray to pink and white. The soup will be very thick, almost like stew, when ready to serve.

Per Serving

calories: 275 | fat: 5g | protein: 18g
carbs: 41g | fiber: 6g | sodium: 644mg

Chicken Provençal Soup

Prep time: 20 minutes | Cook time: 30 minutes | Serves 6 to 8

Ingredients:

1 tablespoon extra-virgin olive oil
2 fennel bulbs, 2 tablespoons fronds minced, stalks discarded, bulbs halved, cored, and cut into ½-inch pieces
1 onion, chopped
1¾ teaspoons table salt
2 tablespoons tomato paste
4 garlic cloves, minced
1 tablespoon minced fresh thyme or 1 teaspoon dried
2 anchovy fillets, minced
7 cups water, divided
1 (14½-ounce / 411-g) can diced tomatoes, drained
2 carrots, peeled, halved lengthwise, and sliced ½ inch thick
2 (12-ounce / 340-g) bone-in split chicken breasts, trimmed
4 (5- to 7-ounce / 142- to 198-g) bone-in chicken thighs, trimmed
½ cup pitted brine-cured green olives, chopped
1 teaspoon grated orange zest

Directions:

1. Using highest sauté function, heat oil in Instant Pot until shimmering. Add fennel pieces, onion, and salt and cook until vegetables are softened, about 5 minutes. Stir in tomato paste, garlic, thyme, and anchovies and cook until fragrant, about 30 seconds. Stir in 5 cups water, scraping up any browned bits, then stir in tomatoes and carrots. Nestle chicken breasts and thighs in pot.
2. Lock lid in place and close pressure release valve. Select high pressure cook function and cook for 20 minutes. Turn off Instant Pot and quick-release pressure. Carefully remove lid, allowing steam to escape away from you.
3. Transfer chicken to cutting board, let cool slightly, then shred into bite-size pieces using 2 forks; discard skin and bones.
4. Using wide, shallow spoon, skim excess fat from surface of soup. Stir chicken and any accumulated juices, olives, and remaining 2 cups water into soup and let sit until heated through, about 3 minutes. Stir in fennel fronds and orange zest, and season with salt and pepper to taste. Serve.

Per Serving

calories: 170 | fat: 5g | protein: 19g
carbs: 11g | fiber: 3g | sodium: 870mg

Israeli Salad

Prep time: 15 minutes | Cook time: 6 minutes | Serves 4

Ingredients:

¼ cup pine nuts
¼ cup shelled pistachios
¼ cup coarsely chopped walnuts
¼ cup shelled pumpkin seeds
¼ cup shelled sunflower seeds
2 large English cucumbers, unpeeled and finely chopped
1 pint cherry tomatoes, finely chopped
½ small red onion, finely chopped
½ cup finely chopped fresh flat-leaf Italian parsley
¼ cup extra-virgin olive oil
2 to 3 tablespoons freshly squeezed lemon juice (from 1 lemon)
1 teaspoon salt
¼ teaspoon freshly ground black pepper
4 cups baby arugula

Directions:

1. In a large dry skillet, toast the pine nuts, pistachios, walnuts, pumpkin seeds, and sunflower seeds over medium-low heat until golden and fragrant, 5 to 6 minutes, being careful not to burn them. Remove from the heat and set aside.
2. In a large bowl, combine the cucumber, tomatoes, red onion, and parsley.
3. In a small bowl, whisk together olive oil, lemon juice, salt, and pepper. Pour over the chopped vegetables and toss to coat.
4. Add the toasted nuts and seeds and arugula and toss with the salad to blend well. Serve at room temperature or chilled.

Per Serving

calories: 414 | fat: 34g | protein: 10g
carbs: 17g | fiber: 6g | sodium: 642mg

Mushroom Barley Soup

Prep time: 5 minutes | Cook time: 25 minutes | Serves 6

Ingredients:

2 tablespoons extra-virgin olive oil
1 cup chopped onion (about ½ medium onion)
1 cup chopped carrots (about 2 carrots)
5½ cups chopped mushrooms (about 12 ounces / 340 g)
6 cups low-sodium or no-salt-added

vegetable broth
1 cup uncooked pearled barley
¼ cup red wine
2 tablespoons tomato paste
4 sprigs fresh thyme or ½ teaspoon dried thyme
1 dried bay leaf
6 tablespoons grated Parmesan cheese

Directions:

1. In a large stockpot over medium heat, heat the oil. Add the onion and carrots and cook for 5 minutes, stirring frequently. Turn up the heat to medium-high and add the mushrooms. Cook for 3 minutes, stirring frequently.
2. Add the broth, barley, wine, tomato paste, thyme, and bay leaf. Stir, cover the pot, and bring the soup to a boil. Once it's boiling, stir a few times, reduce the heat to medium-low, cover, and cook for another 12 to 15 minutes, until the barley is cooked through.
3. Remove the bay leaf and serve in soup bowls with 1 tablespoon of cheese sprinkled on top of each.

Per Serving

calories: 195 | fat: 4g | protein: 7g
carbs: 34g | fiber: 6g | sodium: 173mg

Tomato Hummus Soup

Prep time: 10 minutes | Cook time: 10 minutes | Serves 2

Ingredients:

1 (14½-ounce / 411-g) can crushed tomatoes with basil
1 cup roasted red pepper hummus
2 cups low-sodium chicken stock
Salt, to taste

¼ cup fresh basil leaves, thinly sliced (optional, for garnish)
Garlic croutons (optional, for garnish)

Directions:

1. Combine the canned tomatoes, hummus, and chicken stock in a blender and blend until smooth. Pour the mixture into a saucepan and bring it to a boil.
2. Season with salt and fresh basil if desired. Serve with garlic croutons as a garnish, if desired.

Per Serving

calories: 148 | fat: 6g | protein: 5g
carbs: 19g | fiber: 4g | sodium: 680mg

Pastina Chicken Soup

Prep time: 5 minutes | Cook time: 25 minutes | Serves 6

Ingredients:

1 tablespoon extra-virgin olive oil
2 garlic cloves, minced (about 1 teaspoon)
3 cups packed chopped kale (center ribs removed)
1 cup minced carrots (about 2 carrots)
8 cups low-sodium or no-salt-added chicken (or vegetable) broth

¼ teaspoon kosher or sea salt
¼ teaspoon freshly ground black pepper
¾ cup (6 ounces / 170 g) uncooked acini de pepe or pastina pasta
2 cups shredded cooked chicken (about 12 ounces / 340 g)
3 tablespoons grated Parmesan cheese

Directions:

1. In a large stockpot over medium heat, heat the oil. Add the garlic and cook for 30 seconds, stirring frequently. Add the kale and carrots and cook for 5 minutes, stirring occasionally.
2. Add the broth, salt, and pepper, and turn the heat to high. Bring the broth to a boil, and add the pasta. Lower the heat to medium and cook for 10 minutes, or until the pasta is cooked through, stirring every few minutes so the pasta doesn't stick to the bottom. Add the chicken, and cook for 2 more minutes to warm through.
3. Ladle the soup into six bowls, top each with ½ tablespoon of cheese, and serve.

Per Serving

calories: 275 | fat: 19g | protein: 16g
carbs: 11g | fiber: 2g | sodium: 298mg

Thyme Carrot Soup with Parmesan

Prep time: 10 minutes | Cook time: 20 minutes | Serves 4

Ingredients:

2 pounds (907 g) carrots, unpeeled, cut into ½-inch slices (about 6 cups)
2 tablespoons extra-virgin olive oil, divided
1 cup chopped onion (about ½ medium onion)
2 cups low-sodium or no-salt-added vegetable (or chicken) broth
2½ cups water
1 teaspoon dried thyme
¼ teaspoon crushed red pepper
¼ teaspoon kosher or sea salt
4 thin slices whole-grain bread
⅓ cup freshly grated Parmesan cheese (about 1 ounce / 28 g)

Directions:

1. Place one oven rack about four inches below the broiler element. Place two large, rimmed baking sheets in the oven on any oven rack. Preheat the oven to 450ºF (235ºC).
2. In a large bowl, toss the carrots with 1 tablespoon of oil to coat. With oven mitts, carefully remove the baking sheets from the oven and evenly distribute the carrots on both sheets. Bake for 20 minutes, until the carrots are just fork tender, stirring once halfway through. The carrots will still be somewhat firm. Remove the carrots from the oven, and turn the oven to the high broil setting.
3. While the carrots are roasting, in a large stockpot over medium-high heat, heat 1 tablespoon of oil. Add the onion and cook for 5 minutes, stirring occasionally. Add the broth, water, thyme, crushed red pepper, and salt. Bring to a boil, cover, then remove the pan from the heat until the carrots have finished roasting.
4. Add the roasted carrots to the pot, and blend with an immersion blender (or use a regular blender—carefully pour in the hot soup in batches, then return the soup to the pot). Heat the soup for about 1 minute over medium-high heat, until warmed through.
5. Turn the oven to the high broil setting. Place the bread on the baking sheet. Sprinkle the cheese evenly across the slices of bread. Broil the bread 4 inches below the heating element for 1 to 2 minutes, or until the cheese melts, watching carefully to prevent burning.
6. Cut the bread into bite-size croutons. Divide the soup evenly among four bowls, top each with the Parmesan croutons, and serve.

Per Serving

calories: 312 | fat: 6g | protein: 6g | carbs: 53g | fiber: 10g | sodium: 650mg

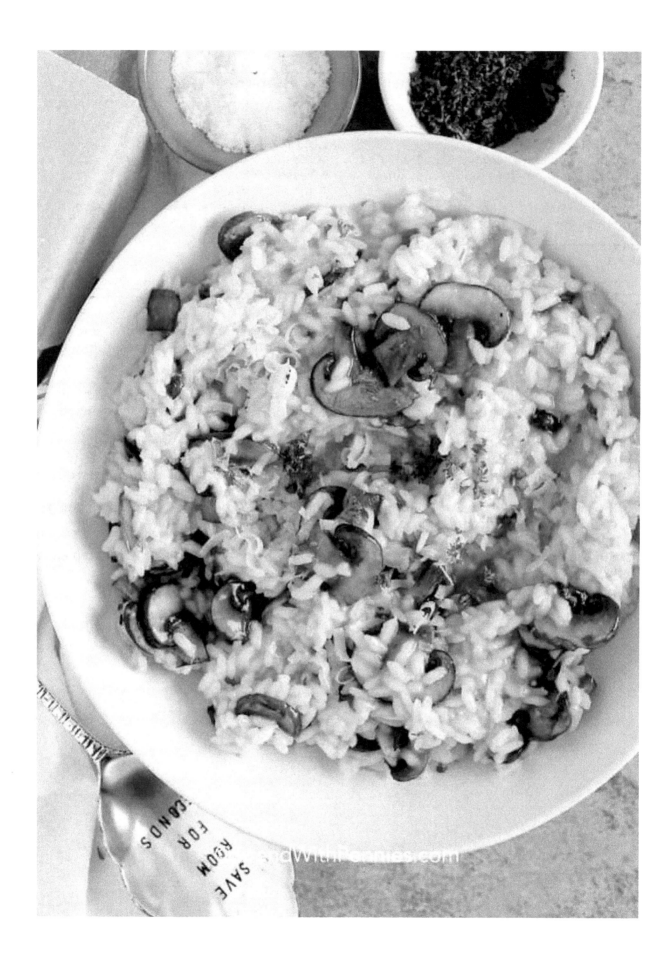

Chapter 5 Beans and Grains

Brown Rice Bowls with Roasted Vegetables

Prep time: 15 minutes | Cook time: 20 minutes | Serves 4

Ingredients:

Nonstick cooking spray
2 cups broccoli florets
2 cups cauliflower florets
1 (15-ounce / 425-g) can chickpeas, drained and rinsed
1 cup carrots sliced 1 inch thick

2 to 3 tablespoons extra-virgin olive oil, divided
Salt and freshly ground black pepper, to taste
2 to 3 tablespoons sesame seeds, for garnish
2 cups cooked brown rice

Dressing:

3 to 4 tablespoons tahini
2 tablespoons honey
1 lemon, juiced
1 garlic clove,

minced
Salt and freshly ground black pepper, to taste

Directions:

1. Preheat the oven to 400ºF (205ºC). Spray two baking sheets with cooking spray.
2. Cover the first baking sheet with the broccoli and cauliflower and the second with the chickpeas and carrots. Toss each sheet with half of the oil and season with salt and pepper before placing in oven.
3. Cook the carrots and chickpeas for 10 minutes, leaving the carrots still just crisp, and the broccoli and cauliflower for 20 minutes, until tender. Stir each halfway through cooking.
4. To make the dressing, in a small bowl, mix the tahini, honey, lemon juice, and garlic. Season with salt and pepper and set aside.
5. Divide the rice into individual bowls, then layer with vegetables and drizzle dressing over the dish.

Per Serving

calories: 454 | fat: 18g | protein: 12g
carbs: 62g | fiber: 11g | sodium: 61mg

Mushroom Parmesan Risotto

Prep time: 10 minutes | Cook time: 30 minutes | Serves 4

Ingredients:

6 cups vegetable broth
3 tablespoons extra-virgin olive oil, divided
1 pound (454 g) cremini mushrooms, cleaned and sliced
1 medium onion,

finely chopped
2 cloves garlic, minced
1½ cups Arborio rice
1 teaspoon salt
½ cup freshly grated Parmesan cheese
½ teaspoon freshly ground black pepper

Directions:

1. In a saucepan over medium heat, bring the broth to a low simmer.
2. In a large skillet over medium heat, cook 1 tablespoon olive oil and the sliced mushrooms for 5 to 7 minutes. Set cooked mushrooms aside.
3. In the same skillet over medium heat, add the 2 remaining tablespoons of olive oil, onion, and garlic. Cook for 3 minutes.
4. Add the rice, salt, and 1 cup of broth to the skillet. Stir the ingredients together and cook over low heat until most of the liquid is absorbed. Continue adding ½ cup of broth at a time, stirring until it is absorbed. Repeat until all of the broth is used up.
5. With the final addition of broth, add the cooked mushrooms, Parmesan cheese, and black pepper. Cook for 2 more minutes. Serve immediately.

Per Serving

calories: 410 | fat: 12g | protein: 11g
carbs: 65g | fiber: 3g | sodium: 2086mg

Lentil Bulgur Pilaf

Prep time: 10 minutes | Cook time: 50 minutes | Serves 6

Ingredients:

½ cup extra-virgin olive oil

4 large onions, chopped

2 teaspoons salt, divided

6 cups water

2 cups brown lentils, picked over and rinsed

1 teaspoon freshly ground black pepper

1 cup bulgur wheat

Directions:

1. In a large pot over medium heat, cook and stir the olive oil, onions, and 1 teaspoon of salt for 12 to 15 minutes, until the onions are a medium brown/golden color.
2. Put half of the cooked onions in a bowl.
3. Add the water, remaining 1 teaspoon of salt, and lentils to the remaining onions. Stir. Cover and cook for 30 minutes.
4. Stir in the black pepper and bulgur, cover, and cook for 5 minutes. Fluff with a fork, cover, and let stand for another 5 minutes.
5. Spoon the lentils and bulgur onto a serving plate and top with the reserved onions. Serve warm.

Per Serving

calories: 479 | fat: 20g | protein: 20g
carbs: 60g | fiber: 24g | sodium: 789mg

Garbanzo and Pita Casserole

Prep time: 10 minutes | Cook time: 10 minutes | Serves 4

Ingredients:

4 cups Greek yogurt

3 cloves garlic, minced

1 teaspoon salt

2 (16-ounce / 454-g) cans garbanzo

beans, rinsed and drained

2 cups water

4 cups pita chips

5 tablespoons unsalted butter

Directions:

1. In a large bowl, whisk together the yogurt, garlic, and salt. Set aside.
2. Put the garbanzo beans and water in a medium pot. Bring to a boil; let beans boil for about 5 minutes.
3. Pour the garbanzo beans and the liquid into a large casserole dish.
4. Top the beans with pita chips. Pour the yogurt sauce over the pita chip layer.
5. In a small saucepan, melt and brown the butter, about 3 minutes. Pour the brown butter over the yogurt sauce.

Per Serving

calories: 772 | fat: 36g | protein: 39g
carbs: 73g | fiber: 13g | sodium: 1003mg

Lentil Stuffed Tomatoes

Prep time: 10 minutes | Cook time: 15 minutes | Serves 4

Ingredients:

4 tomatoes

½ cup cooked red lentils

1 garlic clove, minced

1 tablespoon minced red onion

4 basil leaves, minced

¼ teaspoon salt

¼ teaspoon black pepper

4 ounces (113 g) goat cheese

2 tablespoons shredded Parmesan cheese

Directions:

1. Preheat the air fryer to 380ºF (193ºC).
2. Slice the top off of each tomato.
3. Using a knife and spoon, cut and scoop out half of the flesh inside of the tomato. Place it into a medium bowl.
4. To the bowl with the tomato, add the cooked lentils, garlic, onion, basil, salt, pepper, and goat cheese. Stir until well combined.
5. Spoon the filling into the scooped-out cavity of each of the tomatoes, then top each one with ½ tablespoon of shredded Parmesan cheese.
6. Place the tomatoes in a single layer in the air fryer basket and bake for 15 minutes.

Per Serving

calories: 138 | fat: 7g | protein: 9g
carbs: 11g | fiber: 4g | sodium: 317mg

Baked Sweet Potato Black Bean Burgers

Prep time: 10 minutes | Cook time: 10 minutes | Serves 4

Ingredients:

1 (15-ounce / 425-g) can black beans, drained and rinsed
1 cup mashed sweet potato
½ teaspoon dried oregano
¼ teaspoon dried thyme
¼ teaspoon dried marjoram
1 garlic clove, minced
¼ teaspoon salt
¼ teaspoon black pepper

1 tablespoon lemon juice
1 cup cooked brown rice
¼ to ½ cup whole wheat bread crumbs
1 tablespoon olive oil
For Serving:
Whole wheat buns or whole wheat pitas
Plain Greek yogurt
Avocado
Lettuce
Tomato
Red onion

Directions:

1. Preheat the air fryer to 380ºF (193ºC).
2. In a large bowl, use the back of a fork to mash the black beans until there are no large pieces left.
3. Add the mashed sweet potato, oregano, thyme, marjoram, garlic, salt, pepper, and lemon juice, and mix until well combined.
4. Stir in the cooked rice.
5. Add in ¼ cup of the whole wheat bread crumbs and stir. Check to see if the mixture is dry enough to form patties. If it seems too wet and loose, add an additional ¼ cup bread crumbs and stir.
6. Form the dough into 4 patties. Place them into the air fryer basket in a single layer, making sure that they don't touch each other.
7. Brush half of the olive oil onto the patties and bake for 5 minutes.
8. Flip the patties over, brush the other side with the remaining oil, and bake for an additional 4 to 5 minutes.
9. Serve on toasted whole wheat buns or whole wheat pitas with a spoonful of yogurt and avocado, lettuce, tomato, and red onion as desired.

Per Serving

calories: 263 | fat: 5g | protein: 9g
carbs: 47g | fiber: 8g | sodium: 247mg

Oregano Lentil and Carrot Patties

Prep time: 15 minutes | Cook time: 10 minutes | Serves 4

Ingredients:

1 cup cooked brown lentils
¼ cup fresh parsley leaves
½ cup shredded carrots
¼ red onion, minced
¼ red bell pepper, minced
1 jalapeño, seeded and minced
2 garlic cloves, minced
1 egg
2 tablespoons lemon

juice
2 tablespoons olive oil, divided
½ teaspoon onion powder
½ teaspoon smoked paprika
½ teaspoon dried oregano
¼ teaspoon salt
¼ teaspoon black pepper
½ cup whole wheat bread crumbs

For Serving:

Whole wheat buns or whole wheat pitas
Plain Greek yogurt

Tomato
Lettuce
Red Onion

Directions:

1. Preheat the air fryer to 380ºF (193ºC).
2. In a food processor, pulse the lentils and parsley mostly smooth. (You will want some bits of lentils in the mixture.)
3. Pour the lentils into a large bowl, and combine with the carrots, onion, bell pepper, jalapeño, garlic, egg, lemon juice, and 1 tablespoon olive oil.
4. Add the onion powder, paprika, oregano, salt, pepper, and bread crumbs. Stir everything together until the seasonings and bread crumbs are well distributed.
5. Form the dough into 4 patties. Place them into the air fryer basket in a single layer, making sure that they don't touch each other. Brush the remaining 1 tablespoon of olive oil over the patties.
6. Bake for 5 minutes. Flip the patties over and bake for an additional 5 minutes.
7. Serve on toasted whole wheat buns or whole wheat pitas with a spoonful of yogurt and lettuce, tomato, and red onion as desired.

Per Serving

calories: 206 | fat: 9g | protein: 8g
carbs: 25g | fiber: 6g | sodium: 384mg

Spanish Chicken and Rice

Prep time: 15 minutes | Cook time: 30 minutes | Serves 2

Ingredients:

2 teaspoons smoked paprika
2 teaspoons ground cumin
1½ teaspoons garlic salt
¾ teaspoon chili powder
¼ teaspoon dried oregano
1 lemon
2 boneless, skinless chicken breasts
3 tablespoons extra-virgin olive oil, divided
2 large shallots, diced
1 cup uncooked white rice
2 cups vegetable stock
1 cup broccoli florets
⅓ cup chopped parsley

Directions:

1. In a small bowl, whisk together the paprika, cumin, garlic salt, chili powder, and oregano. Divide in half and set aside. Into another small bowl, juice the lemon and set aside.
2. Put the chicken in a medium bowl. Coat the chicken with 2 tablespoons of olive oil and rub with half of the seasoning mix.
3. In a large pan, heat the remaining 1 tablespoon of olive oil and cook the chicken for 2 to 3 minutes on each side, until just browned but not cooked through.
4. Add shallots to the same pan and cook until translucent, then add the rice and cook for 1 more minute to toast. Add the vegetable stock, lemon juice, and the remaining seasoning mix and stir to combine. Return the chicken to the pan on top of the rice. Cover and cook for 15 minutes.
5. Uncover and add the broccoli florets. Cover and cook an additional 5 minutes, until the liquid is absorbed, rice is tender, and chicken is cooked through.
6. Top with freshly chopped parsley and serve immediately.

Per Serving

calories: 750 | fat: 25g | protein: 36g
carbs: 101g | fiber: 7g | sodium: 1823mg

Mushroom Barley Pilaf

Prep time: 5 minutes | Cook time: 37 minutes | Serves 4

Ingredients:

Olive oil cooking spray
2 tablespoons olive oil
8 ounces (227 g) button mushrooms, diced
½ yellow onion, diced
2 garlic cloves, minced
1 cup pearl barley
2 cups vegetable broth
1 tablespoon fresh thyme, chopped
½ teaspoon salt
¼ teaspoon smoked paprika
Fresh parsley, for garnish

Directions:

1. Preheat the air fryer to 380ºF (193ºC). Lightly coat the inside of a 5-cup capacity casserole dish with olive oil cooking spray. (The shape of the casserole dish will depend upon the size of the air fryer, but it needs to be able to hold at least 5 cups.)
2. In a large skillet, heat the olive oil over medium heat. Add the mushrooms and onion and cook, stirring occasionally, for 5 minutes, or until the mushrooms begin to brown.
3. Add the garlic and cook for an additional 2 minutes. Transfer the vegetables to a large bowl.
4. Add the barley, broth, thyme, salt, and paprika.
5. Pour the barley-and-vegetable mixture into the prepared casserole dish, and place the dish into the air fryer. Bake for 15 minutes.
6. Stir the barley mixture. Reduce the heat to 360ºF (182ºC), then return the barley to the air fryer and bake for 15 minutes more.
7. Remove from the air fryer and let sit for 5 minutes before fluffing with a fork and topping with fresh parsley.

Per Serving

calories: 263 | fat: 8g | protein: 7g
carbs: 44g | fiber: 9g | sodium: 576mg

Creamy Parmesan Garlic Polenta

Prep time: 5 minutes | Cook time: 30 minutes | Serves 4

Ingredients:

4 tablespoons (½ stick) unsalted butter, divided
1 tablespoon garlic, finely chopped

4 cups water
1 teaspoon salt
1 cup polenta
¾ cup Parmesan cheese, divided

Directions:

1. In a large pot over medium heat, cook 3 tablespoons of butter and the garlic for 2 minutes.
2. Add the water and salt, and bring to a boil. Add the polenta and immediately whisk until it starts to thicken, about 3 minutes. Turn the heat to low, cover, and cook for 25 minutes, whisking every 5 minutes.
3. Using a wooden spoon, stir in ½ cup of the Parmesan cheese.
4. To serve, pour the polenta into a large serving bowl. Sprinkle the top with the remaining 1 tablespoon butter and ¼ cup of remaining Parmesan cheese. Serve warm.

Per Serving

calories: 297 | fat: 16g | protein: 9g
carbs: 28g | fiber: 2g | sodium: 838mg

Herb Lentil-Rice Balls

Prep time: 5 minutes | Cook time: 11 minutes | Serves 6

Ingredients:

½ cup cooked green lentils
2 garlic cloves, minced
¼ white onion, minced
¼ cup parsley leaves

5 basil leaves
1 cup cooked brown rice
1 tablespoon lemon juice
1 tablespoon olive oil
½ teaspoon salt

Directions:

1. Preheat the air fryer to 380ºF (193ºC).
2. In a food processor, pulse the cooked lentils with the garlic, onion, parsley, and basil until mostly smooth. (You will want some bits of lentils in the mixture.)
3. Pour the lentil mixture into a large bowl, and stir in brown rice, lemon juice, olive oil, and salt. Stir until well combined.
4. Form the rice mixture into 1-inch balls. Place the rice balls in a single layer in the air fryer basket, making sure that they don't touch each other.
5. Fry for 6 minutes. Turn the rice balls and then fry for an additional 4 to 5 minutes, or until browned on all sides.
6. **Per Serving**

calories: 80 | fat: 3g | protein: 2g
carbs: 12g | fiber: 2g | sodium: 198mg

Rustic Lentil-Rice Pilaf

Prep time: 5 minutes | Cook time: 50 minutes | Serves 6

Ingredients:

¼ cup extra-virgin olive oil
1 large onion, chopped
6 cups water
1 teaspoon ground

cumin
1 teaspoon salt
2 cups brown lentils, picked over and rinsed
1 cup basmati rice

Directions:

1. In a medium pot over medium heat, cook the olive oil and onions for 7 to 10 minutes until the edges are browned.
2. Turn the heat to high, add the water, cumin, and salt, and bring this mixture to a boil, boiling for about 3 minutes.
3. Add the lentils and turn the heat to medium-low. Cover the pot and cook for 20 minutes, stirring occasionally.
4. Stir in the rice and cover; cook for an additional 20 minutes.
5. Fluff the rice with a fork and serve warm.

Per Serving

calories: 397 | fat: 11g | protein: 18g
carbs: 60g | fiber: 18g | sodium: 396mg

Bulgur Pilaf with Garbanzos

Prep time: 5 minutes | Cook time: 20 minutes | Serves 4 to 6

Ingredients:

3 tablespoons extra-virgin olive oil
1 large onion, chopped
1 (16-ounce / 454-g) can garbanzo beans, rinsed and drained
2 cups bulgur wheat, rinsed and drained
1½ teaspoons salt
½ teaspoon cinnamon
4 cups water

Directions:

1. In a large pot over medium heat, cook the olive oil and onion for 5 minutes.
2. Add the garbanzo beans and cook for another 5 minutes.
3. Add the bulgur, salt, cinnamon, and water and stir to combine. Cover the pot, turn the heat to low, and cook for 10 minutes.
4. When the cooking is done, fluff the pilaf with a fork. Cover and let sit for another 5 minutes.

Per Serving

calories: 462 | fat: 13g | protein: 15g
carbs: 76g | fiber: 19g | sodium: 890mg

Simple Spanish Rice

Prep time: 10 minutes | Cook time: 20 minutes | Serves 4

Ingredients:

2 tablespoons extra-virgin olive oil
1 medium onion, finely chopped
1 large tomato, finely diced
2 tablespoons
tomato paste
1 teaspoon smoked paprika
1 teaspoon salt
1½ cups basmati rice
3 cups water

Directions:

1. In a medium pot over medium heat, cook the olive oil, onion, and tomato for 3 minutes.
2. Stir in the tomato paste, paprika, salt, and rice. Cook for 1 minute.
3. Add the water, cover the pot, and turn the heat to low. Cook for 12 minutes.
4. Gently toss the rice, cover, and cook for another 3 minutes.

Per Serving

calories: 328 | fat: 7g | protein: 6g
carbs: 60g | fiber: 2g | sodium: 651mg

Orzo Vegetable Pilaf

Prep time: 20 minutes | Cook time: 10 minutes | Serves 6

Ingredients:

2 cups orzo
1 pint (2 cups) cherry tomatoes, cut in half
1 cup Kalamata olives
½ cup fresh basil, finely chopped
½ cup extra-virgin olive oil
⅓ cup balsamic vinegar
1 teaspoon salt
½ teaspoon freshly ground black pepper

Directions:

1. Bring a large pot of water to a boil. Add the orzo and cook for 7 minutes. Drain and rinse the orzo with cold water in a strainer.
2. Once the orzo has cooled, put it in a large bowl. Add the tomatoes, olives, and basil.
3. In a small bowl, whisk together the olive oil, vinegar, salt, and pepper. Add this dressing to the pasta and toss everything together. Serve at room temperature or chilled.

Per Serving

calories: 476 | fat: 28g | protein: 8g
carbs: 48g | fiber: 3g | sodium: 851mg

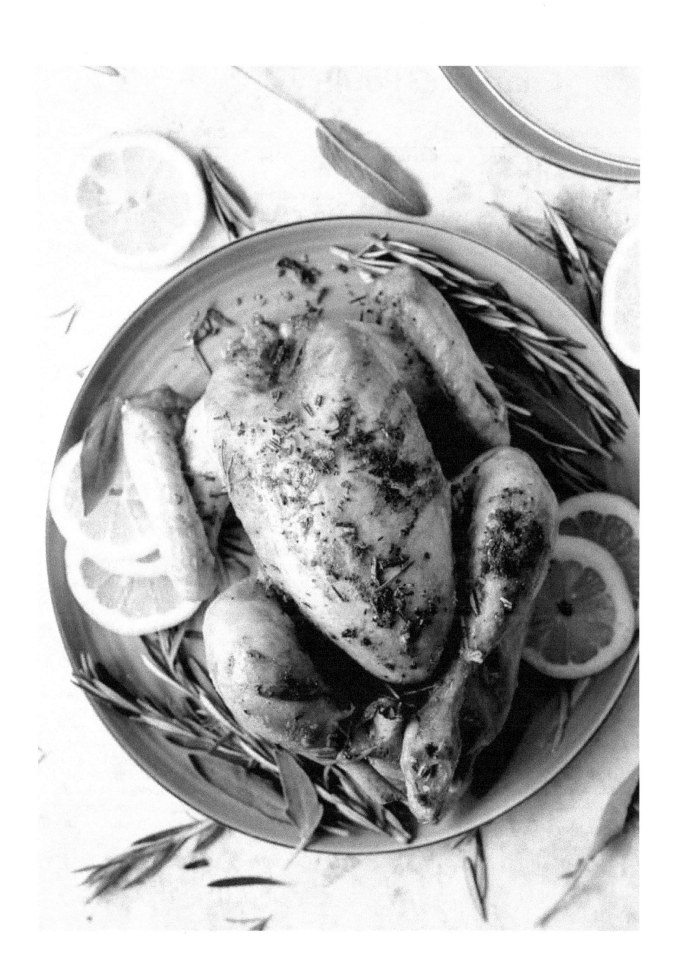

Chapter 6 Poultry and Meats

Feta Stuffed Chicken Breasts

Prep time: 10 minutes | Cook time: 20 minutes | Serves 4

Ingredients:

$1/_3$ cup cooked brown rice
1 teaspoon shawarma seasoning
4 (6-ounce / 170-g) boneless skinless chicken breasts
1 tablespoon harissa
3 tablespoons extra-virgin olive oil, divided
Salt and freshly ground black pepper, to taste
4 small dried apricots, halved
$1/_3$ cup crumbled feta
1 tablespoon chopped fresh parsley

Directions:

1. Preheat the oven to 375ºF (190ºC).
2. In a medium bowl, mix the rice and shawarma seasoning and set aside.
3. Butterfly the chicken breasts by slicing them almost in half, starting at the thickest part and folding them open like a book.
4. In a small bowl, mix the harissa with 1 tablespoon of olive oil. Brush the chicken with the harissa oil and season with salt and pepper. The harissa adds a nice heat, so feel free to add a thicker coating for more spice.
5. Onto one side of each chicken breast, spoon 1 to 2 tablespoons of rice, then layer 2 apricot halves in each breast. Divide the feta between the chicken breasts and fold the other side over the filling to close.
6. In an oven-safe sauté pan or skillet, heat the remaining 2 tablespoons of olive oil and sear the breast for 2 minutes on each side, then place the pan into the oven for 15 minutes, or until fully cooked and juices run clear. Serve, garnished with parsley.

Per Serving

calories: 321 | fat: 17g | protein: 37g
carbs: 8g | fiber: 1g | sodium: 410mg

Greek Lemon Chicken Kebabs

Prep time: 15 minutes | Cook time: 20 minutes | Serves 2

Ingredients:

½ cup extra-virgin olive oil, divided
½ large lemon, juiced
2 garlic cloves, minced
½ teaspoon za'atar seasoning
Salt and freshly ground black pepper, to taste
1 pound (454 g) boneless skinless chicken breasts, cut into 1¼-inch cubes
1 large red bell pepper, cut into 1¼-inch pieces
2 small zucchini (nearly 1 pound / 454 g), cut into rounds slightly under ½ inch thick
2 large shallots, diced into quarters
Tzatziki sauce, for serving

Directions:

1. In a bowl, whisk together $1/_3$ cup of olive oil, lemon juice, garlic, za'atar, salt, and pepper.
2. Put the chicken in a medium bowl and pour the olive oil mixture over the chicken. Press the chicken into the marinade. Cover and refrigerate for 45 minutes. While the chicken marinates, soak the wooden skewers in water for 30 minutes.
3. Drizzle and toss the pepper, zucchini, and shallots with the remaining 2½ tablespoons of olive oil and season lightly with salt.
4. Preheat the oven to 500ºF (260ºC) and put a baking sheet in the oven to heat.
5. On each skewer, thread a red bell pepper, zucchini, shallot and 2 chicken pieces and repeat twice. Put the kebabs onto the hot baking sheet and cook for 7 to 9 minutes, or until the chicken is cooked through. Rotate once halfway through cooking. Serve the kebabs warm with the tzatziki sauce.

Per Serving (2 kebabs)

calories: 825 | fat: 59g | protein: 51g
carbs: 31g | fiber: 5g | sodium: 379mg

Greek-Style Lamb Burgers

Prep time: 10 minutes | Cook time: 10 minutes | Serves 4

Ingredients:

1 pound (454 g) ground lamb
½ teaspoon salt
½ teaspoon freshly ground black pepper

4 tablespoons feta cheese, crumbled
Buns, toppings, and tzatziki, for serving (optional)

Directions:

1. Preheat a grill, grill pan, or lightly oiled skillet to high heat.
2. In a large bowl, using your hands, combine the lamb with the salt and pepper.
3. Divide the meat into 4 portions. Divide each portion in half to make a top and a bottom. Flatten each half into a 3-inch circle. Make a dent in the center of one of the halves and place 1 tablespoon of the feta cheese in the center. Place the second half of the patty on top of the feta cheese and press down to close the 2 halves together, making it resemble a round burger.
4. Cook the stuffed patty for 3 minutes on each side, for medium-well. Serve on a bun with your favorite toppings and tzatziki sauce, if desired.

Per Serving

calories: 345 | fat: 29g | protein: 20g
carbs: 1g | fiber: 0g | sodium: 462mg

Lemon-Rosemary Lamb Chops

Prep time: 10 minutes | Cook time: 10 minutes | Serves 6

Ingredients:

4 large cloves garlic
1 cup lemon juice
1/3 cup fresh rosemary
1 cup extra-virgin olive oil

1½ teaspoons salt
1 teaspoon freshly ground black pepper
6 (1-inch-thick) lamb chops

Directions:

1. In a food processor or blender, blend the garlic, lemon juice, rosemary, olive oil, salt, and black pepper for 15 seconds. Set aside.

2. Put the lamb chops in a large plastic zip-top bag or container. Cover the lamb with two-thirds of the rosemary dressing, making sure that all of the lamb chops are coated with the dressing. Let the lamb marinate in the fridge for 1 hour.
3. When you are almost ready to eat, take the lamb chops out of the fridge and let them sit on the counter-top for 20 minutes. Preheat a grill, grill pan, or lightly oiled skillet to high heat.
4. Cook the lamb chops for 3 minutes on each side. To serve, drizzle the lamb with the remaining dressing.

Per Serving

calories: 484 | fat: 42g | protein: 24g
carbs: 5g | fiber: 1g | sodium: 655mg

Braised Veal Shanks

Prep time: 10 minutes | Cook time: 2 hours | Serves 4

Ingredients:

4 veal shanks, bone in
½ cup flour
4 tablespoons extra-virgin olive oil
1 large onion, chopped
5 cloves garlic, sliced

2 teaspoons salt
1 tablespoon fresh thyme
3 tablespoons tomato paste
6 cups water
Cooked noodles, for serving (optional)

Directions:

1. Preheat the oven to 350ºF (180ºC).
2. Dredge the veal shanks in the flour.
3. Pour the olive oil into a large oven-safe pot or pan over medium heat; add the veal shanks. Brown the veal on both sides, about 4 minutes each side. Remove the veal from pot and set aside.
4. Add the onion, garlic, salt, thyme, and tomato paste to the pan and cook for 3 to 4 minutes. Add the water, and stir to combine.
5. Add the veal back to the pan, and bring to a simmer. Cover the pan with a lid or foil and bake for 1 hour and 50 minutes. Remove from the oven and serve with cooked noodles, if desired.

Per Serving

calories: 400 | fat: 19g | protein: 39g
carbs: 18g | fiber: 2g | sodium: 1368mg

Lamb Koftas with Lime Yogurt Sauce

Prep time: 30 minutes | Cook time: 15 minutes | Serves 4

Ingredients:

1 pound (454 g) ground lamb
½ cup finely chopped fresh mint, plus 2 tablespoons
¼ cup almond or coconut flour
¼ cup finely chopped red onion
¼ cup toasted pine nuts
2 teaspoons ground cumin
1½ teaspoons salt, divided

1 teaspoon ground cinnamon
1 teaspoon ground ginger
½ teaspoon ground nutmeg
½ teaspoon freshly ground black pepper
1 cup plain whole-milk Greek yogurt
2 tablespoons extra-virgin olive oil
Zest and juice of 1 lime

Directions:

1. Heat the oven broiler to the low setting. You can also bake these at high heat (450 to 475ºF / 235 to 245ºC) if you happen to have a very hot broiler. Submerge four wooden skewers in water and let soak at least 10 minutes to prevent them from burning.
2. In a large bowl, combine the lamb, ½ cup mint, almond flour, red onion, pine nuts, cumin, 1 teaspoon salt, cinnamon, ginger, nutmeg, and pepper and, using your hands, incorporate all the ingredients together well.
3. Form the mixture into 12 egg-shaped patties and let sit for 10 minutes.
4. Remove the skewers from the water, thread 3 patties onto each skewer, and place on a broiling pan or wire rack on top of a baking sheet lined with aluminum foil. Broil on the top rack until golden and cooked through, 8 to 12 minutes, flipping once halfway through cooking.
5. While the meat cooks, in a small bowl, combine the yogurt, olive oil, remaining 2 tablespoons chopped mint, remaining ½ teaspoon salt, and lime zest and juice and whisk to combine well. Keep cool until ready to use.
6. Serve the skewers with yogurt sauce.

Per Serving

calories: 500 | fat: 42g | protein: 23g
carbs: 9g | fiber: 2g | sodium: 969mg

Braised Garlic Flank Steak with Artichokes

Prep time: 15 minutes | Cook time: 60 minutes | Serves 4 to 6

Ingredients:

4 tablespoons grapeseed oil, divided
2 pounds (907 g) flank steak
1 (14-ounce / 397-g) can artichoke hearts, drained and roughly chopped
1 onion, diced
8 garlic cloves, chopped
1 (32-ounce / 907-g) container low-sodium beef broth
1 (14½-ounce /

411-g) can diced tomatoes, drained
1 cup tomato sauce
2 tablespoons tomato paste
1 teaspoon dried oregano
1 teaspoon dried parsley
1 teaspoon dried basil
½ teaspoon ground cumin
3 bay leaves
2 to 3 cups cooked couscous (optional)

Directions:

1. Preheat the oven to 450ºF (235ºC).
2. In an oven-safe sauté pan or skillet, heat 3 tablespoons of oil on medium heat. Sear the steak for 2 minutes per side on both sides. Transfer the steak to the oven for 30 minutes, or until desired tenderness.
3. Meanwhile, in a large pot, combine the remaining 1 tablespoon of oil, artichoke hearts, onion, and garlic. Pour in the beef broth, tomatoes, tomato sauce, and tomato paste. Stir in oregano, parsley, basil, cumin, and bay leaves.
4. Cook the vegetables, covered, for 30 minutes. Remove bay leaf and serve with flank steak and ½ cup of couscous per plate, if using.

Per Serving

calories: 577 | fat: 28g | protein: 55g
carbs: 22g | fiber: 6g | sodium: 1405mg

Spatchcock Chicken with Lemon and Rosemary

Prep time: 20 minutes | Cook time: 45 minutes | Serves 6 to 8

Ingredients:

½ cup extra-virgin olive oil, divided
1 (3- to 4-pound / 1.4- to 1.8-kg) roasting chicken
8 garlic cloves, roughly chopped
2 to 4 tablespoons chopped fresh rosemary
2 teaspoons salt, divided
1 teaspoon freshly ground black pepper, divided
2 lemons, thinly sliced

Directions:

1. Preheat the oven to 425ºF (220ºC).
2. Pour 2 tablespoons olive oil in the bottom of a 9-by-13-inch baking dish or rimmed baking sheet and swirl to coat the bottom.
3. To spatchcock the bird, place the whole chicken breast-side down on a large work surface. Using a very sharp knife, cut along the backbone, starting at the tail end and working your way up to the neck. Pull apart the two sides, opening up the chicken. Flip it over, breast-side up, pressing down with your hands to flatten the bird. Transfer to the prepared baking dish.
4. Loosen the skin over the breasts and thighs by cutting a small incision and sticking one or two fingers inside to pull the skin away from the meat without removing it.
5. To prepare the filling, in a small bowl, combine ¼ cup olive oil, garlic, rosemary, 1 teaspoon salt, and ½ teaspoon pepper and whisk together.
6. Rub the garlic-herb oil evenly under the skin of each breast and each thigh. Add the lemon slices evenly to the same areas.
7. Whisk together the remaining 2 tablespoons olive oil, 1 teaspoon salt, and ½ teaspoon pepper and rub over the outside of the chicken.
8. Place in the oven, uncovered, and roast for 45 minutes, or until cooked through and golden brown. Allow to rest 5 minutes before carving to serve.

Per Serving

calories: 435 | fat: 34g | protein: 28g
carbs: 2g | fiber: 0g | sodium: 879mg

Lemon Chicken Thighs with Vegetables

Prep time: 15 minutes | Cook time: 45 minutes | Serves 4

Ingredients:

6 tablespoons extra-virgin olive oil, divided
4 large garlic cloves, crushed
1 tablespoon dried basil
1 tablespoon dried parsley
1 tablespoon salt
½ tablespoon thyme
4 skin-on, bone-in chicken thighs
6 medium portobello mushrooms, quartered
1 large zucchini, sliced
1 large carrot, thinly sliced
⅛ cup pitted Kalamata olives
8 pieces sun-dried tomatoes (optional)
½ cup dry white wine
1 lemon, sliced

Directions:

1. In a small bowl, combine 4 tablespoons of olive oil, the garlic cloves, basil, parsley, salt, and thyme. Store half of the marinade in a jar and, in a bowl, combine the remaining half to marinate the chicken thighs for about 30 minutes.
2. Preheat the oven to 425ºF (220ºC).
3. In a large skillet or oven-safe pan, heat the remaining 2 tablespoons of olive oil over medium-high heat. Sear the chicken for 3 to 5 minutes on each side until golden brown, and set aside.
4. In the same pan, sauté portobello mushrooms, zucchini, and carrot for about 5 minutes, or until lightly browned.
5. Add the chicken thighs, olives, and sun-dried tomatoes (if using). Pour the wine over the chicken thighs.
6. Cover the pan and cook for about 10 minutes over medium-low heat.
7. Uncover the pan and transfer it to the oven. Cook for 15 more minutes, or until the chicken skin is crispy and the juices run clear. Top with lemon slices.

Per Serving

calories: 544 | fat: 41g | protein: 28g
carbs: 20g | fiber: 11g | sodium: 1848mg

Traditional Chicken Shawarma

Prep time: 15 minutes | Cook time: 15 minutes | Serves 4 to 6

Ingredients:

2 pounds (907 g) boneless and skinless chicken
½ cup lemon juice
½ cup extra-virgin olive oil
3 tablespoons minced garlic
1½ teaspoons salt
½ teaspoon freshly ground black pepper
½ teaspoon ground cardamom
½ teaspoon cinnamon
Hummus and pita bread, for serving (optional)

Directions:

1. Cut the chicken into ¼-inch strips and put them into a large bowl.
2. In a separate bowl, whisk together the lemon juice, olive oil, garlic, salt, pepper, cardamom, and cinnamon.
3. Pour the dressing over the chicken and stir to coat all of the chicken.
4. Let the chicken sit for about 10 minutes.
5. Heat a large pan over medium-high heat and cook the chicken pieces for 12 minutes, using tongs to turn the chicken over every few minutes.
6. Serve with hummus and pita bread, if desired.

Per Serving

calories: 477 | fat: 32g | protein: 47g
carbs: 5g | fiber: 1g | sodium: 1234mg

Chicken Shish Tawook

Prep time: 15 minutes | Cook time: 15 minutes | Serves 4 to 6

Ingredients:

2 tablespoons garlic, minced
2 tablespoons tomato paste
1 teaspoon smoked paprika
½ cup lemon juice
½ cup extra-virgin olive oil
1½ teaspoons salt
½ teaspoon freshly ground black pepper
2 pounds (907 g) boneless and skinless chicken (breasts or thighs)
Rice, tzatziki, or hummus, for serving (optional)

Directions:

1. In a large bowl, add the garlic, tomato paste, paprika, lemon juice, olive oil, salt, and pepper and whisk to combine.
2. Cut the chicken into ½-inch cubes and put them into the bowl; toss to coat with the marinade. Set aside for at least 10 minutes.
3. To grill, preheat the grill on high. Thread the chicken onto skewers and cook for 3 minutes per side, for a total of 9 minutes.
4. To cook in a pan, preheat the pan on high heat, add the chicken, and cook for 9 minutes, turning over the chicken using tongs.
5. Serve the chicken with rice, tzatziki, or hummus, if desired.

Per Serving

calories: 482 | fat: 32g | protein: 47g
carbs: 6g | fiber: 1g | sodium: 1298mg

Beef Kefta

Prep time: 10 minutes | Cook time: 5 minutes | Serves 4

Ingredients:

1 medium onion
⅓ cup fresh Italian parsley
1 pound (454 g) ground beef
¼ teaspoon ground cumin
¼ teaspoon cinnamon
1 teaspoon salt
½ teaspoon freshly ground black pepper

Directions:

1. Preheat a grill or grill pan to high.
2. Mince the onion and parsley in a food processor until finely chopped.
3. In a large bowl, using your hands, combine the beef with the onion mix, ground cumin, cinnamon, salt, and pepper.
4. Divide the meat into 6 portions. Form each portion into a flat oval.
5. Place the patties on the grill or grill pan and cook for 3 minutes on each side.

Per Serving

calories: 203 | fat: 10g | protein: 24g
carbs: 3g | fiber: 1g | sodium: 655mg

Mediterranean Grilled Skirt Steak

Prep time: 10 minutes | Cook time: 10 minutes | Serves 4

Ingredients:

1 pound (454 g) skirt steak
1 teaspoon salt
½ teaspoon freshly ground black pepper

2 cups prepared hummus
1 tablespoon extra-virgin olive oil
½ cup pine nuts

Directions:

1. Preheat a grill, grill pan, or lightly oiled skillet to medium heat.
2. Season both sides of the steak with salt and pepper.
3. Cook the meat on each side for 3 to 5 minutes; 3 minutes for medium, and 5 minutes on each side for well done. Let the meat rest for 5 minutes.
4. Slice the meat into thin strips.
5. Spread the hummus on a serving dish, and evenly distribute the beef on top of the hummus.
6. In a small saucepan, over low heat, add the olive oil and pine nuts. Toast them for 3 minutes, constantly stirring them with a spoon so that they don't burn.
7. Spoon the pine nuts over the beef and serve.

Per Serving

calories: 602 | fat: 41g | protein: 42g
carbs: 20g | fiber: 8g | sodium: 1141mg

Pork Souvlaki with Oregano

Prep time: 10 minutes | Cook time: 10 minutes | Serves 4

Ingredients:

1 (1½-pound / 680-g) pork loin
2 tablespoons garlic, minced
⅓ cup extra-virgin olive oil
⅓ cup lemon juice

1 tablespoon dried oregano
1 teaspoon salt
Pita bread and tzatziki, for serving (optional)

Directions:

1. Cut the pork into 1-inch cubes and put them into a bowl or plastic zip-top bag.
2. In a large bowl, mix together the garlic, olive oil, lemon juice, oregano, and salt.
3. Pour the marinade over the pork and let it marinate for at least 1 hour.
4. Preheat a grill, grill pan, or lightly oiled skillet to high heat. Using wood or metal skewers, thread the pork onto the skewers.
5. Cook the skewers for 3 minutes on each side, for 12 minutes in total.
6. Serve with pita bread and tzatziki sauce, if desired.

Per Serving

calories: 416 | fat: 30g | protein: 32g
carbs: 5g | fiber: 1g | sodium: 1184mg

Moroccan Chicken Meatballs

Prep time: 10 minutes | Cook time: 10 minutes | Serves 4 to 6

Ingredients:

2 large shallots, diced
2 tablespoons finely chopped parsley
2 teaspoons paprika
1 teaspoon ground cumin
½ teaspoon ground coriander
½ teaspoon garlic powder

½ teaspoon salt
½ teaspoon freshly ground black pepper
⅛ teaspoon ground cardamom
1 pound (454 g) ground chicken
½ cup all-purpose flour, to coat
¼ cup olive oil, divided

Directions:

1. In a bowl, combine the shallots, parsley, paprika, cumin, coriander, garlic powder, salt, pepper, and cardamom. Mix well.
2. Add the chicken to the spice mixture and mix well. Form into 1-inch balls flattened to about ½-inch thickness.
3. Put the flour in a bowl for dredging. Dip the balls into the flour until coated.
4. Pour enough oil to cover the bottom of a sauté pan or skillet and heat over medium heat. Working in batches, cook the meatballs, turning frequently, for 2 to 3 minutes on each side, until they are cooked through. Add more oil between batches as needed. Serve in a pita, topped with lettuce dressed with Creamy Yogurt Dressing.

Per Serving

calories: 405 | fat: 26g | protein: 24g
carbs: 20g | fiber: 1g | sodium: 387mg

Chicken Skewers with Veggies

Prep time: 30 minutes | Cook time: 25 minutes | Serves 4

Ingredients:

¼ cup olive oil
1 teaspoon garlic powder
1 teaspoon onion powder
1 teaspoon ground cumin
½ teaspoon dried oregano
½ teaspoon dried basil
¼ cup lemon juice
1 tablespoon apple cider vinegar

Olive oil cooking spray
1 pound (454 g) boneless skinless chicken thighs, cut into 1-inch pieces
1 red bell pepper, cut into 1-inch pieces
1 red onion, cut into 1-inch pieces
1 zucchini, cut into 1-inch pieces
12 cherry tomatoes

Directions:

1. In a large bowl, mix together the olive
2. oil, garlic powder, onion powder, cumin, oregano, basil, lemon juice, and apple cider vinegar.
3. Spray six skewers with olive oil cooking spray.
4. On each skewer, slide on a piece of chicken, then a piece of bell pepper, onion, zucchini, and finally a tomato and then repeat. Each skewer should have at least two pieces of each item.
5. Once all of the skewers are prepared, place them in a 9-by-13-inch baking dish and pour the olive oil marinade over the top of the skewers. Turn each skewer so that all sides of the chicken and vegetables are coated.
6. Cover the dish with plastic wrap and place it in the refrigerator for 30 minutes.
7. After 30 minutes, preheat the air fryer to 380ºF (193ºC). (If using a grill attachment, make sure it is inside the air fryer during preheating.)
8. Remove the skewers from the marinade and lay them in a single layer in the air fryer basket. If the air fryer has a grill attachment, you can also lay them on this instead.
9. Cook for 10 minutes. Rotate the kebabs, then cook them for 15 minutes more.
10. Remove the skewers from the air fryer and let them rest for 5 minutes before serving.

Per Serving

calories: 304 | fat: 17g | protein: 27g
carbs: 10g | fiber: 3g | sodium: 62mg

Moroccan Pot Roast

Prep time: 15 minutes | Cook time: 50 minutes | Serves 4

Ingredients:

8 ounces (227 g) mushrooms, sliced
4 tablespoons extra-virgin olive oil
3 small onions, cut into 2-inch pieces
2 tablespoons paprika
1½ tablespoons garam masala
2 teaspoons salt
¼ teaspoon ground white pepper
2 tablespoons tomato paste

1 small eggplant, peeled and diced
1¼ cups low-sodium beef broth
½ cup halved apricots
⅓ cup golden raisins
3 pounds (1.4 kg) beef chuck roast
2 tablespoons honey
1 tablespoon dried mint
2 cups cooked brown rice

Directions:

1. Set an electric pressure cooker to Sauté and put the mushrooms and oil in the cooker. Sauté for 5 minutes, then add the onions, paprika, garam masala, salt, and white pepper. Stir in the tomato paste and continue to sauté.
2. Add the eggplant and sauté for 5 more minutes, until softened. Pour in the broth. Add the apricots and raisins. Sear the meat for 2 minutes on each side.
3. Close and lock the lid and set the pressure cooker to high for 50 minutes.
4. When cooking is complete, quick release the pressure. Carefully remove the lid, then remove the meat from the sauce and break it into pieces. While the meat is removed, stir honey and mint into the sauce.
5. Assemble plates with ½ cup of brown rice, ½ cup of pot roast sauce, and 3 to 5 pieces of pot roast.

Per Serving

calories: 829 | fat: 34g | protein: 69g
carbs: 70g | fiber: 11g | sodium: 1556mg

Grilled Beef Kebabs

Prep time: 15 minutes | Cook time: 10 minutes | Serves 6

Ingredients:

2 pounds (907 g) beef fillet
1½ teaspoons salt
1 teaspoon freshly ground black pepper
½ teaspoon ground allspice
½ teaspoon ground nutmeg
⅓ cup extra-virgin olive oil
1 large onion, cut into 8 quarters
1 large red bell pepper, cut into 1-inch cubes

Directions:

1. Preheat a grill, grill pan, or lightly oiled skillet to high heat.
2. Cut the beef into 1-inch cubes and put them in a large bowl.
3. In a small bowl, mix together the salt, black pepper, allspice, and nutmeg.
4. Pour the olive oil over the beef and toss to coat the beef. Then evenly sprinkle the seasoning over the beef and toss to coat all pieces.
5. Skewer the beef, alternating every 1 or 2 pieces with a piece of onion or bell pepper.
6. To cook, place the skewers on the grill or skillet, and turn every 2 to 3 minutes until all sides have cooked to desired doneness, 6 minutes for medium-rare, 8 minutes for well done. Serve warm.

Per Serving

calories: 485 | fat: 36g | protein: 35g | carbs: 4g | fiber: 1g | sodium: 1453mg

Lemon-Garlic Whole Chicken and Potatoes

Prep time: 10 minutes | Cook time: 45 minutes | Serves 4 to 6

Ingredients:

1 cup garlic, minced
1½ cups lemon juice
1 cup plus 2 tablespoons extra-virgin olive oil, divided
1½ teaspoons salt, divided
1 teaspoon freshly ground black pepper
1 whole chicken, cut into 8 pieces
1 pound (454 g) fingerling or red potatoes

Directions:

1. Preheat the oven to 400ºF (205ºC).
2. In a large bowl, whisk together the garlic, lemon juice, 1 cup of olive oil, 1 teaspoon of salt, and pepper.
3. Put the chicken in a large baking dish and pour half of the lemon sauce over the chicken. Cover the baking dish with foil, and cook for 20 minutes.
4. Cut the potatoes in half, and toss to coat with 2 tablespoons olive oil and 1 teaspoon of salt. Put them on a baking sheet and bake for 20 minutes in the same oven as the chicken.
5. Take both the chicken and potatoes out of the oven. Using a spatula, transfer the potatoes to the baking dish with the chicken. Pour the remaining sauce over the potatoes and chicken. Bake for another 25 minutes.
6. Transfer the chicken and potatoes to a serving dish and spoon the garlic-lemon sauce from the pan on top.

Per Serving

calories: 959 | fat: 78g | protein: 33g | carbs: 37g | fiber: 4g | sodium: 1005mg

Yogurt-Marinated Chicken

Prep time: 15 minutes | Cook time: 30 minutes | Serves 2

Ingredients:

½ cup plain Greek yogurt
3 garlic cloves, minced
2 tablespoons minced fresh oregano (or 1 tablespoon dried oregano)
Zest of 1 lemon

1 tablespoon olive oil
½ teaspoon salt
2 (4-ounce / 113-g) boneless, skinless chicken breasts

Directions:

1. In a medium bowl, add the yogurt, garlic, oregano, lemon zest, olive oil, and salt and stir to combine. If the yogurt is very thick, you may need to add a few tablespoons of water or a squeeze of lemon juice to thin it a bit.
2. Add the chicken to the bowl and toss it in the marinade to coat it well. Cover and refrigerate the chicken for at least 30 minutes or up to overnight.
3. Preheat the oven to 350ºF (180ºC) and set the rack to the middle position.
4. Place the chicken in a baking dish and roast for 30 minutes, or until chicken reaches an internal temperature of 165ºF (74ºC).

Per Serving

calories: 255 | fat: 13g | protein: 29g | carbs: 8g | fiber: 2g | sodium: 694mg

Beef and Potatoes with Tahini Sauce

Prep time: 10 minutes | Cook time: 30 minutes | Serves 4 to 6

Ingredients:

1 pound (454 g) ground beef
2 teaspoons salt, divided
½ teaspoon freshly ground black pepper
1 large onion, finely chopped
10 medium golden potatoes

2 tablespoons extra-virgin olive oil
3 cups Greek yogurt
1 cup tahini
3 cloves garlic, minced
2 cups water

Directions:

1. Preheat the oven to 450ºF (235ºC).
2. In a large bowl, using your hands, combine the beef with 1 teaspoon salt, black pepper, and the onion.
3. Form meatballs of medium size (about 1-inch), using about 2 tablespoons of the beef mixture. Place them in a deep 8-by-8-inch casserole dish.
4. Cut the potatoes into ¼-inch-thick slices. Toss them with the olive oil.
5. Lay the potato slices flat on a lined baking sheet.
6. Put the baking sheet with the potatoes and the casserole dish with the meatballs in the oven and bake for 20 minutes.
7. In a large bowl, mix together the yogurt, tahini, garlic, remaining 1 teaspoon salt, and water; set aside.
8. Once you take the meatballs and potatoes out of the oven, use a spatula to transfer the potatoes from the baking sheet to the casserole dish with the meatballs, and leave the beef drippings in the casserole dish for added flavor.
9. Reduce the oven temperature to 375ºF (190ºC) and pour the yogurt tahini sauce over the beef and potatoes. Return it to the oven for 10 minutes. Once baking is complete, serve warm with a side of rice or pita bread.

Per Serving

calories: 1078 | fat: 59g | protein: 58g | carbs: 89g | fiber: 11g | sodium: 1368mg

Mediterranean Lamb Bowls

Prep time: 15 minutes | Cook time: 15 minutes | Serves 2

Ingredients:

2 tablespoons extra-virgin olive oil
¼ cup diced yellow onion
1 pound (454 g) ground lamb
1 teaspoon dried mint
1 teaspoon dried parsley
½ teaspoon red pepper flakes
¼ teaspoon garlic powder

1 cup cooked rice
½ teaspoon za'atar seasoning
½ cup halved cherry tomatoes
1 cucumber, peeled and diced
1 cup store-bought hummus
1 cup crumbled feta cheese
2 pita breads, warmed (optional)

Directions:

1. In a large sauté pan or skillet, heat the olive oil over medium heat and cook the onion for about 2 minutes, until fragrant. Add the lamb and mix well, breaking up the meat as you cook. Once the lamb is halfway cooked, add mint, parsley, red pepper flakes, and garlic powder.
2. In a medium bowl, mix together the cooked rice and za'atar, then divide between individual serving bowls. Add the seasoned lamb, then top the bowls with the tomatoes, cucumber, hummus, feta, and pita (if using).

Per Serving

calories: 1312 | fat: 96g | protein: 62g | carbs: 62g | fiber: 12g | sodium: 1454mg

Herbed Lamb Burgers

Prep time: 15 minutes | Cook time: 15 minutes | Serves 4

Ingredients:

1 pound (454 g) ground lamb
½ small red onion, grated
1 tablespoon dried parsley
1 teaspoon dried oregano
1 teaspoon ground cumin
1 teaspoon garlic powder
½ teaspoon dried mint

¼ teaspoon paprika
¼ teaspoon kosher salt
⅛ teaspoon freshly ground black pepper
Extra-virgin olive oil
4 pita breads, for serving (optional)
Tzatziki sauce, for serving (optional)
Pickled onions, for serving (optional)

Directions:

1. In a bowl, combine the lamb, onion, parsley, oregano, cumin, garlic powder, mint, paprika, salt, and pepper. Divide the meat into 4 small balls and work into smooth discs.
2. In a large sauté pan or skillet, heat a drizzle of olive oil over medium heat or brush a grill with oil and set it to medium. Cook the patties for 4 to 5 minutes on each side, until cooked through and juices run clear.
3. Enjoy lamb burgers in pitas, topped with tzatziki sauce and pickled onions (if using).

Per Serving

calories: 328 | fat: 27g | protein: 19g | carbs: 2g | fiber: 1g | sodium: 215mg

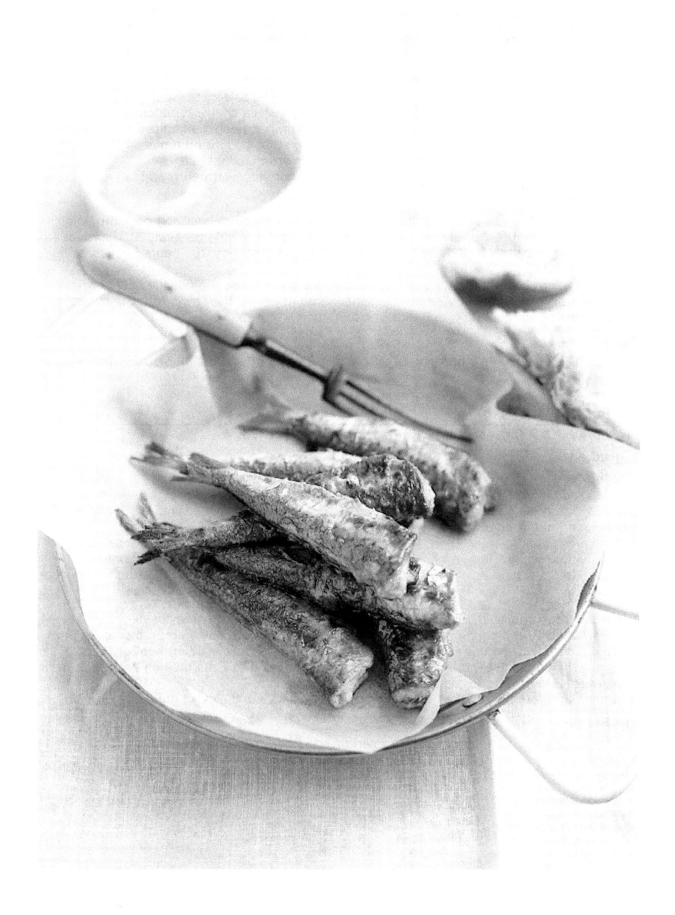

Chapter 7 Fish and Seafood

Grilled Lemon Shrimp

Prep time: 20 minutes | Cook time: 5 minutes | Serves 4 to 6

Ingredients:

2 tablespoons garlic, minced
½ cup lemon juice
3 tablespoons fresh Italian parsley, finely chopped
¼ cup extra-virgin

olive oil
1 teaspoon salt
2 pounds (907 g) jumbo shrimp (21 to 25), peeled and deveined

Directions:

1. In a large bowl, mix the garlic, lemon juice, parsley, olive oil, and salt.
2. Add the shrimp to the bowl and toss to make sure all the pieces are coated with the marinade. Let the shrimp sit for 15 minutes.
3. Preheat a grill, grill pan, or lightly oiled skillet to high heat. While heating, thread about 5 to 6 pieces of shrimp onto each skewer.
4. Place the skewers on the grill, grill pan, or skillet and cook for 2 to 3 minutes on each side until cooked through. Serve warm.

Per Serving

calories: 402 | fat: 18g | protein: 57g
carbs: 4g | fiber: 0g | sodium: 1224mg

Italian Fried Shrimp

Prep time: 10 minutes | Cook time: 5 minutes | Serves 4

Ingredients:

2 large eggs
2 cups seasoned Italian bread crumbs
1 teaspoon salt
1 cup flour

1 pound (454 g) large shrimp (21 to 25), peeled and deveined
Extra-virgin olive oil

Directions:

1. In a small bowl, beat the eggs with 1 tablespoon water, then transfer to a shallow dish.

2. Add the bread crumbs and salt to a separate shallow dish; mix well.
3. Place the flour into a third shallow dish.
4. Coat the shrimp in the flour, then egg, and finally the bread crumbs. Place on a plate and repeat with all of the shrimp.
5. Preheat a skillet over high heat. Pour in enough olive oil to coat the bottom of the skillet. Cook the shrimp in the hot skillet for 2 to 3 minutes on each side. Take the shrimp out and drain on a paper towel. Serve warm.

Per Serving

calories: 714 | fat: 34g | protein: 37g
carbs: 63g | fiber: 3g | sodium: 1727mg

Crispy Fried Sardines

Prep time: 5 minutes | Cook time: 5 minutes | Serves 4

Ingredients:

Avocado oil, as needed
1½ pounds (680 g) whole fresh sardines, scales removed

1 teaspoon salt
1 teaspoon freshly ground black pepper
2 cups flour

Directions:

1. Preheat a deep skillet over medium heat. Pour in enough oil so there is about 1 inch of it in the pan.
2. Season the fish with the salt and pepper.
3. Dredge the fish in the flour so it is completely covered.
4. Slowly drop in 1 fish at a time, making sure not to overcrowd the pan.
5. Cook for about 3 minutes on each side or just until the fish begins to brown on all sides. Serve warm.

Per Serving

calories: 794 | fat: 47g | protein: 48g
carbs: 44g | fiber: 2g | sodium: 1441mg

Cod Saffron Rice

Prep time: 10 minutes | Cook time: 35 minutes | Serves 4

Ingredients:

4 tablespoons extra-virgin olive oil, divided
1 large onion, chopped
3 cod fillets, rinsed and patted dry
4½ cups water
1 teaspoon saffron threads
1½ teaspoons salt
1 teaspoon turmeric
2 cups long-grain rice, rinsed

Directions:

1. In a large pot over medium heat, cook 2 tablespoons of olive oil and the onions for 5 minutes.
2. While the onions are cooking, preheat another large pan over high heat. Add the remaining 2 tablespoons of olive oil and the cod fillets. Cook the cod for 2 minutes on each side, then remove from the pan and set aside.
3. Once the onions are done cooking, add the water, saffron, salt, turmeric, and rice, stirring to combine. Cover and cook for 12 minutes.
4. Cut the cod up into 1-inch pieces. Place the cod pieces in the rice, lightly toss, cover, and cook for another 10 minutes.
5. Once the rice is done cooking, fluff with a fork, cover, and let stand for 5 minutes. Serve warm.

Per Serving

calories: 564 | fat: 15g | protein: 26g
carbs: 78g | fiber: 2g | sodium: 945mg

Thyme Whole Roasted Red Snapper

Prep time: 5 minutes | Cook time: 45 minutes | Serves 4

Ingredients:

1 (2 to 2½ pounds / 907 g to 1.1 kg) whole red snapper, cleaned and scaled
2 lemons, sliced (about 10 slices)
3 cloves garlic, sliced
4 or 5 sprigs of thyme
3 tablespoons cold salted butter, cut into small cubes, divided

Directions:

1. Preheat the oven to 350ºF (180ºC).

2. Cut a piece of foil to about the size of your baking sheet; put the foil on the baking sheet.
3. Make a horizontal slice through the belly of the fish to create a pocket.
4. Place 3 slices of lemon on the foil and the fish on top of the lemons.
5. Stuff the fish with the garlic, thyme, 3 lemon slices and butter. Reserve 3 pieces of butter.
6. Place the reserved 3 pieces of butter on top of the fish, and 3 or 4 slices of lemon on top of the butter. Bring the foil together and seal it to make a pocket around the fish.
7. Put the fish in the oven and bake for 45 minutes. Serve with remaining fresh lemon slices.

Per Serving

calories: 345 | fat: 13g | protein: 54g
carbs: 12g | fiber: 3g | sodium: 170mg

Cilantro Lemon Shrimp

Prep time: 20 minutes | Cook time: 10 minutes | Serves 4

Ingredients:

⅓ cup lemon juice
4 garlic cloves
1 cup fresh cilantro leaves
½ teaspoon ground coriander
3 tablespoons extra-virgin olive oil
1 teaspoon salt
1½ pounds (680 g) large shrimp (21 to 25), deveined and shells removed

Directions:

1. In a food processor, pulse the lemon juice, garlic, cilantro, coriander, olive oil, and salt 10 times.
2. Put the shrimp in a bowl or plastic zip-top bag, pour in the cilantro marinade, and let sit for 15 minutes.
3. Preheat a skillet on high heat.
4. Put the shrimp and marinade in the skillet. Cook the shrimp for 3 minutes on each side. Serve warm.

Per Serving

calories: 225 | fat: 12g | protein: 28g
carbs: 5g | fiber: 1g | sodium: 763mg

Olive Oil-Poached Tuna

Prep time: 5 minutes | Cook time: 45 minutes | Serves 4

Ingredients:

1 cup extra-virgin olive oil, plus more if needed
4 (3- to 4-inch) sprigs fresh rosemary
8 (3- to 4-inch) sprigs fresh thyme
2 large garlic cloves, thinly sliced
2 (2-inch) strips lemon zest
1 teaspoon salt
½ teaspoon freshly ground black pepper
1 pound (454 g) fresh tuna steaks (about 1 inch thick)

Directions:

1. Select a thick pot just large enough to fit the tuna in a single layer on the bottom. The larger the pot, the more olive oil you will need to use. Combine the olive oil, rosemary, thyme, garlic, lemon zest, salt, and pepper over medium-low heat and cook until warm and fragrant, 20 to 25 minutes, lowering the heat if it begins to smoke.
2. Remove from the heat and allow to cool for 25 to 30 minutes, until warm but not hot.
3. Add the tuna to the bottom of the pan, adding additional oil if needed so that tuna is fully submerged, and return to medium-low heat. Cook for 5 to 10 minutes, or until the oil heats back up and is warm and fragrant but not smoking. Lower the heat if it gets too hot.
4. Remove the pot from the heat and let the tuna cook in warm oil 4 to 5 minutes, to your desired level of doneness. For a tuna that is rare in the center, cook for 2 to 3 minutes.
5. Remove from the oil and serve warm, drizzling 2 to 3 tablespoons seasoned oil over the tuna.
6. To store for later use, remove the tuna from the oil and place in a container with a lid. Allow tuna and oil to cool separately. When both have cooled, remove the herb stems with a slotted spoon and pour the cooking oil over the tuna. Cover and store in the refrigerator for up to 1 week. Bring to room temperature to allow the oil to liquify before serving.

Per Serving

calories: 363 | fat: 28g | protein: 27g
carbs: 1g | fiber: 0g | sodium: 624mg

Fideos with Seafood

Prep time: 15 minutes | Cook time: 20 minutes | Serves 6 to 8

Ingredients:

2 tablespoons extra-virgin olive oil, plus ½ cup, divided
6 cups zucchini noodles, roughly chopped (2 to 3 medium zucchini)
1 pound (454 g) shrimp, peeled, deveined and roughly chopped
6 to 8 ounces (170 to 227 g) canned chopped clams, drained
4 ounces (113 g) crab meat
½ cup crumbled goat cheese
½ cup crumbled feta cheese
1 (28-ounce / 794-g) can chopped tomatoes, with their juices
1 teaspoon salt
1 teaspoon garlic powder
½ teaspoon smoked paprika
½ cup shredded Parmesan cheese
¼ cup chopped fresh flat-leaf Italian parsley, for garnish

Directions:

1. Preheat the oven to 375ºF (190ºC).
2. Pour 2 tablespoons olive oil in the bottom of a 9-by-13-inch baking dish and swirl to coat the bottom.
3. In a large bowl, combine the zucchini noodles, shrimp, clams, and crab meat.
4. In another bowl, combine the goat cheese, feta, and ¼ cup olive oil and stir to combine well. Add the canned tomatoes and their juices, salt, garlic powder, and paprika and combine well. Add the mixture to the zucchini and seafood mixture and stir to combine.
5. Pour the mixture into the prepared baking dish, spreading evenly. Spread shredded Parmesan over top and drizzle with the remaining ¼ cup olive oil. Bake until bubbly, 20 to 25 minutes. Serve warm, garnished with chopped parsley.

Per Serving

calories: 434 | fat: 31g | protein: 29g
carbs: 12g | fiber: 3g | sodium: 712mg

Orange Roasted Salmon

Prep time: 10 minutes | Cook time: 25 minutes | Serves 4

Ingredients:

½ cup extra-virgin olive oil, divided
2 tablespoons balsamic vinegar
2 tablespoons garlic powder, divided
1 tablespoon cumin seeds
1 teaspoon sea salt, divided
1 teaspoon freshly ground black pepper, divided
2 teaspoons smoked paprika
4 (8-ounce / 227-g) salmon fillets, skinless
2 small red onion, thinly sliced
½ cup halved Campari tomatoes
1 small fennel bulb, thinly sliced lengthwise
1 large carrot, thinly sliced
8 medium portobello mushrooms
8 medium radishes, sliced ⅛ inch thick
½ cup dry white wine
½ lime, zested
Handful cilantro leaves
½ cup halved pitted Kalamata olives
1 orange, thinly sliced
4 roasted sweet potatoes, cut in wedges lengthwise

Directions:

1. Preheat the oven to 375ºF (190ºC).
2. In a medium bowl, mix 6 tablespoons of olive oil, the balsamic vinegar, 1 tablespoon of garlic powder, the cumin seeds, ¼ teaspoon of sea salt, ¼ teaspoon of pepper, and the paprika. Put the salmon in the bowl and marinate while preparing the vegetables, about 10 minutes.
3. Heat an oven-safe sauté pan or skillet on medium-high heat and sear the top of the salmon for about 2 minutes, or until lightly brown. Set aside.
4. Add the remaining 2 tablespoons of olive oil to the same skillet. Once it's hot, add the onion, tomatoes, fennel, carrot, mushrooms, radishes, the remaining 1 teaspoon of garlic powder, ¾ teaspoon of salt, and ¾ teaspoon of pepper. Mix well and cook for 5 to 7 minutes, until fragrant. Add wine and mix well.
5. Place the salmon on top of the vegetable mixture, browned-side up. Sprinkle the fish with lime zest and cilantro and place the olives around the fish. Put orange slices over the fish and cook for about 7 additional minutes. While this is baking, add the sliced sweet potato wedges on a baking sheet and bake this alongside the skillet.
6. Remove from the oven, cover the skillet tightly, and let rest for about 3 minutes.

Per Serving

calories: 841 | fat: 41g | protein: 59g
carbs: 60g | fiber: 15g | sodium: 908mg

Shrimp with Garlic and Mushrooms

Prep time: 10 minutes | Cook time: 15 minutes | Serves 4

Ingredients:

1 pound (454 g) peeled and deveined fresh shrimp
1 teaspoon salt
1 cup extra-virgin olive oil
8 large garlic cloves, thinly sliced
4 ounces (113 g) sliced mushrooms
(shiitake, baby bella, or button)
½ teaspoon red pepper flakes
¼ cup chopped fresh flat-leaf Italian parsley
Zucchini noodles or riced cauliflower, for serving

Directions:

1. Rinse the shrimp and pat dry. Place in a small bowl and sprinkle with the salt.
2. In a large rimmed, thick skillet, heat the olive oil over medium-low heat. Add the garlic and heat until very fragrant, 3 to 4 minutes, reducing the heat if the garlic starts to burn.
3. Add the mushrooms and sauté for 5 minutes, until softened. Add the shrimp and red pepper flakes and sauté until the shrimp begins to turn pink, another 3 to 4 minutes.
4. Remove from the heat and stir in the parsley. Serve over zucchini noodles or riced cauliflower.

Per Serving

calories: 620 | fat: 56g | protein: 24g
carbs: 4g | fiber: 0g | sodium: 736mg

Seafood Risotto

Prep time: 10 minutes | Cook time: 30 minutes | Serves 4

Ingredients:

6 cups vegetable broth
3 tablespoons extra-virgin olive oil
1 large onion, chopped
3 cloves garlic, minced
½ teaspoon saffron threads
1½ cups arborio rice
1½ teaspoons salt
8 ounces (227 g) shrimp (21 to 25), peeled and deveined
8 ounces (227 g) scallops

Directions:

1. In a large saucepan over medium heat, bring the broth to a low simmer.
2. In a large skillet over medium heat, cook the olive oil, onion, garlic, and saffron for 3 minutes.
3. Add the rice, salt, and 1 cup of the broth to the skillet. Stir the ingredients together and cook over low heat until most of the liquid is absorbed. Repeat steps with broth, adding ½ cup of broth at a time, and cook until all but ½ cup of the broth is absorbed.
4. Add the shrimp and scallops when you stir in the final ½ cup of broth. Cover and let cook for 10 minutes. Serve warm.

Per Serving

calories: 460 | fat: 12g | protein: 24g
carbs: 64g | fiber: 2g | sodium: 2432mg

Garlic Shrimp Black Bean Pasta

Prep time: 10 minutes | Cook time: 15 minutes | Serves 4

Ingredients:

1 pound (454 g) black bean linguine or spaghetti
1 pound (454 g) fresh shrimp, peeled and deveined
4 tablespoons extra-virgin olive oil
1 onion, finely chopped
3 garlic cloves, minced
¼ cup basil, cut into strips

Directions:

1. Bring a large pot of water to a boil and cook the pasta according to the package instructions.

2. In the last 5 minutes of cooking the pasta, add the shrimp to the hot water and allow them to cook for 3 to 5 minutes. Once they turn pink, take them out of the hot water, and, if you think you may have overcooked them, run them under cool water. Set aside.
3. Reserve 1 cup of the pasta cooking water and drain the noodles. In the same pan, heat the oil over medium-high heat and cook the onion and garlic for 7 to 10 minutes. Once the onion is translucent, add the pasta back in and toss well.
4. Plate the pasta, then top with shrimp and garnish with basil.

Per Serving

calories: 668 | fat: 19g | protein: 57g
carbs: 73g | fiber: 31g | sodium: 615mg

Baked Trout with Lemon

Prep time: 5 minutes | Cook time: 15 minutes | Serves 4

Ingredients:

4 trout fillets
2 tablespoons olive oil
½ teaspoon salt
1 teaspoon black pepper
2 garlic cloves, sliced
1 lemon, sliced, plus additional wedges for serving

Directions:

1. Preheat the air fryer to 380ºF (193ºC).
2. Brush each fillet with olive oil on both sides and season with salt and pepper. Place the fillets in an even layer in the air fryer basket.
3. Place the sliced garlic over the tops of the trout fillets, then top the garlic with lemon slices and cook for 12 to 15 minutes, or until it has reached an internal temperature of 145ºF (63ºC).
4. Serve with fresh lemon wedges.

Per Serving

calories: 231 | fat: 12g | protein: 29g
carbs: 1g | fiber: 0g | sodium: 341mg

Fast Seafood Paella

Prep time: 20 minutes | Cook time: 20 minutes | Serves 4

Ingredients:

¼ cup plus 1 tablespoon extra-virgin olive oil
1 large onion, finely chopped
2 tomatoes, peeled and chopped
1½ tablespoons garlic powder
1½ cups medium-grain Spanish paella rice or arborio rice
2 carrots, finely diced
Salt, to taste

1 tablespoon sweet paprika
8 ounces (227 g) lobster meat or canned crab
½ cup frozen peas
3 cups chicken stock, plus more if needed
1 cup dry white wine
6 jumbo shrimp, unpeeled
⅓ pound (136 g) calamari rings
1 lemon, halved

Directions:

1. In a large sauté pan or skillet (16-inch is ideal), heat the oil over medium heat until small bubbles start to escape from oil. Add the onion and cook for about 3 minutes, until fragrant, then add tomatoes and garlic powder. Cook for 5 to 10 minutes, until the tomatoes are reduced by half and the consistency is sticky.
2. Stir in the rice, carrots, salt, paprika, lobster, and peas and mix well. In a pot or microwave-safe bowl, heat the chicken stock to almost boiling, then add it to the rice mixture. Bring to a simmer, then add the wine.
3. Smooth out the rice in the bottom of the pan. Cover and cook on low for 10 minutes, mixing occasionally, to prevent burning.
4. Top the rice with the shrimp, cover, and cook for 5 more minutes. Add additional broth to the pan if the rice looks dried out.
5. Right before removing the skillet from the heat, add the calamari rings. Toss the ingredients frequently. In about 2 minutes, the rings will look opaque. Remove the pan from the heat immediately—you don't want the paella to overcook). Squeeze fresh lemon juice over the dish.

Per Serving

calories: 632 | fat: 20g | protein: 34g
carbs: 71g | fiber: 5g | sodium: 920mg

Classic Escabeche

Prep time: 10 minutes | Cook time: 20 minutes | Serves 4

Ingredients:

1 pound (454 g) wild-caught Spanish mackerel fillets, cut into four pieces
1 teaspoon salt
½ teaspoon freshly ground black pepper
8 tablespoons extra-virgin olive oil, divided
1 bunch asparagus, trimmed and cut into

2-inch pieces
1 (13¾-ounce / 390-g) can artichoke hearts, drained and quartered
4 large garlic cloves, peeled and crushed
2 bay leaves
¼ cup red wine vinegar
½ teaspoon smoked paprika

Directions:

1. Sprinkle the fillets with salt and pepper and let sit at room temperature for 5 minutes.
2. In a large skillet, heat 2 tablespoons olive oil over medium-high heat. Add the fish, skin-side up, and cook 5 minutes. Flip and cook 5 minutes on the other side, until browned and cooked through. Transfer to a serving dish, pour the cooking oil over the fish, and cover to keep warm.
3. Heat the remaining 6 tablespoons olive oil in the same skillet over medium heat. Add the asparagus, artichokes, garlic, and bay leaves and sauté until the vegetables are tender, 6 to 8 minutes.
4. Using a slotted spoon, top the fish with the cooked vegetables, reserving the oil in the skillet. Add the vinegar and paprika to the oil and whisk to combine well. Pour the vinaigrette over the fish and vegetables and let sit at room temperature for at least 15 minutes, or marinate in the refrigerator up to 24 hours for a deeper flavor. Remove the bay leaf before serving.

Per Serving

calories: 578 | fat: 50g | protein: 26g
carbs: 13g | fiber: 5g | sodium: 946mg

Sea Bass Crusted with Moroccan Spices

Prep time: 15 minutes | Cook time: 40 minutes | Serves 4

Ingredients:

1½ teaspoons ground turmeric, divided
¾ teaspoon saffron
½ teaspoon ground cumin
¼ teaspoon kosher salt
¼ teaspoon freshly ground black pepper
1½ pounds (680 g) sea bass fillets, about ½ inch thick
8 tablespoons extra-virgin olive oil, divided
8 garlic cloves, divided (4 minced cloves and 4 sliced)
6 medium baby portobello mushrooms, chopped
1 large carrot, sliced on an angle
2 sun-dried tomatoes, thinly sliced (optional)
2 tablespoons tomato paste
1 (15-ounce / 425-g) can chickpeas, drained and rinsed
1½ cups low-sodium vegetable broth
¼ cup white wine
1 tablespoon ground coriander (optional)
1 cup sliced artichoke hearts marinated in olive oil
½ cup pitted Kalamata olives
½ lemon, juiced
½ lemon, cut into thin rounds
4 to 5 rosemary sprigs or 2 tablespoons dried rosemary
Fresh cilantro, for garnish

Directions:

1. In a small mixing bowl, combine 1 teaspoon turmeric and the saffron and cumin. Season with salt and pepper. Season both sides of the fish with the spice mixture. Add 3 tablespoons of olive oil and work the fish to make sure it's well coated with the spices and the olive oil.
2. In a large sauté pan or skillet, heat 2 tablespoons of olive oil over medium heat until shimmering but not smoking. Sear the top side of the sea bass for about 1 minute, or until golden. Remove and set aside.
3. In the same skillet, add the minced garlic and cook very briefly, tossing regularly, until fragrant. Add the mushrooms, carrot, sun-dried tomatoes (if using), and tomato paste. Cook for 3 to 4 minutes over medium heat, tossing frequently, until fragrant. Add the chickpeas, broth, wine, coriander (if using), and the sliced garlic. Stir in the remaining ½ teaspoon ground turmeric. Raise the heat, if needed, and bring to a boil, then lower heat to simmer. Cover part of the way and let the sauce simmer for about 20 minutes, until thickened.
4. Carefully add the seared fish to the skillet. Ladle a bit of the sauce on top of the fish. Add the artichokes, olives, lemon juice and slices, and rosemary sprigs. Cook another 10 minutes or until the fish is fully cooked and flaky. Garnish with fresh cilantro.

Per Serving

calories:696 | fat: 41g | protein: 48g
carbs: 37g | fiber: 9g | sodium: 810mg

Shrimp Pesto Rice Bowls

Prep time: 5 minutes | Cook time: 5 minutes | Serves 4

Ingredients:

1 pound (454 g) medium shrimp, peeled and deveined
¼ cup pesto sauce
1 lemon, sliced
2 cups cooked wild rice pilaf

Directions:

1. Preheat the air fryer to 360ºF (182ºC).
2. In a medium bowl, toss the shrimp with the pesto sauce until well coated.
3. Place the shrimp in a single layer in the air fryer basket. Put the lemon slices over the shrimp and roast for 5 minutes.
4. Remove the lemons and discard. Serve a quarter of the shrimp over ½ cup wild rice with some favorite steamed vegetables.

Per Serving

calories: 249 | fat: 10g | protein: 20g
carbs: 20g | fiber: 2g | sodium: 277mg

Lemon Rosemary Branzino

Prep time: 15 minutes | Cook time: 30 minutes | Serves 2

Ingredients:

4 tablespoons extra-virgin olive oil, divided
2 (8-ounce / 227-g) branzino fillets, preferably at least 1 inch thick
1 garlic clove, minced
1 bunch scallions, white part only, thinly sliced
½ cup sliced pitted Kalamata or other good-quality black olives
1 large carrot, cut into ¼-inch rounds

10 to 12 small cherry tomatoes, halved
½ cup dry white wine
2 tablespoons paprika
2 teaspoons kosher salt
½ tablespoon ground chili pepper, preferably Turkish or Aleppo
2 rosemary sprigs or 1 tablespoon dried rosemary
1 small lemon, very thinly sliced

Directions:

1. Warm a large, oven-safe sauté pan or skillet over high heat until hot, about 2 minutes. Carefully add 1 tablespoon of olive oil and heat until it shimmers, 10 to 15 seconds. Brown the branzino fillets for 2 minutes, skin-side up. Carefully flip the fillets skin-side down and cook for another 2 minutes, until browned. Set aside.
2. Swirl 2 tablespoons of olive oil around the skillet to coat evenly. Add the garlic, scallions, kalamata olives, carrot, and tomatoes, and let the vegetables sauté for 5 minutes, until softened. Add the wine, stirring until all ingredients are well integrated. Carefully place the fish over the sauce.
3. Preheat the oven to 450ºF (235ºC).
4. While the oven is heating, brush the fillets with 1 tablespoon of olive oil and season with paprika, salt, and chili pepper. Top each fillet with a rosemary sprig and several slices of lemon. Scatter the olives over fish and around the pan.
5. Roast until lemon slices are browned or singed, about 10 minutes.

Per Serving

calories: 725 | fat: 43g | protein: 58g | carbs: 25g | fiber: 10g | sodium: 2954mg

Almond-Crusted Swordfish

Prep time: 25 minutes | Cook time: 15 minutes | Serves 4

Ingredients:

½ cup almond flour
¼ cup crushed Marcona almonds
½ to 1 teaspoon salt, divided
2 pounds (907 g) Swordfish, preferably 1 inch thick
1 large egg, beaten (optional)
¼ cup pure apple cider
¼ cup extra-virgin olive oil, plus more for frying

3 to 4 sprigs flat-leaf parsley, chopped
1 lemon, juiced
1 tablespoon Spanish paprika
5 medium baby portobello mushrooms, chopped (optional)
4 or 5 chopped scallions, both green and white parts
3 to 4 garlic cloves, peeled
¼ cup chopped pitted Kalamata olives

Directions:

1. On a dinner plate, spread the flour and crushed Marcona almonds and mix in the salt. Alternately, pour the flour, almonds, and ¼ teaspoon of salt into a large plastic food storage bag. Add the fish and coat it with the flour mixture. If a thicker coat is desired, repeat this step after dipping the fish in the egg (if using).
2. In a measuring cup, combine the apple cider, ¼ cup of olive oil, parsley, lemon juice, paprika, and ¼ teaspoon of salt. Mix well and set aside.

3. In a large, heavy-bottom sauté pan or skillet, pour the olive oil to a depth of ⅛ inch and heat on medium heat. Once the oil is hot, add the fish and brown for 3 to 5 minutes, then turn the fish over and add the mushrooms (If using), scallions, garlic, and olives. Cook for an additional 3 minutes. Once the other side of the fish is brown, remove the fish from the pan and set aside.
4. Pour the cider mixture into the skillet and mix well with the vegetables. Put the fried fish into the skillet on top of the mixture and cook with sauce on medium-low heat for 10 minutes, until the fish flakes easily with a fork. Carefully remove the fish from the pan and plate. Spoon the sauce over the fish. Serve with white rice or home-fried potatoes.

Per Serving

calories: 620 | fat: 37g | protein: 63g | carbs: 10g | fiber: 5g | sodium: 644mg

Salmon with Tomatoes and Olives

Prep time: 5 minutes | Cook time: 8 minutes | Serves 4

Ingredients:

2 tablespoons olive oil
4 (1½-inch-thick) salmon fillets
½ teaspoon salt
¼ teaspoon cayenne

1 teaspoon chopped fresh dill
2 Roma tomatoes, diced
¼ cup sliced Kalamata olives
4 lemon slices

Directions:

1. Preheat the air fryer to 380ºF (193ºC).
2. Brush the olive oil on both sides of the salmon fillets, and then season them lightly with salt, cayenne, and dill.
3. Place the fillets in a single layer in the basket of the air fryer, then layer the tomatoes and olives over the top. Top each fillet with a lemon slice.
4. Bake for 8 minutes, or until the salmon has reached an internal temperature of 145ºF (63ºC).

Per Serving

calories: 241 | fat: 15g | protein: 23g | carbs: 3g | fiber: 1g | sodium: 595mg

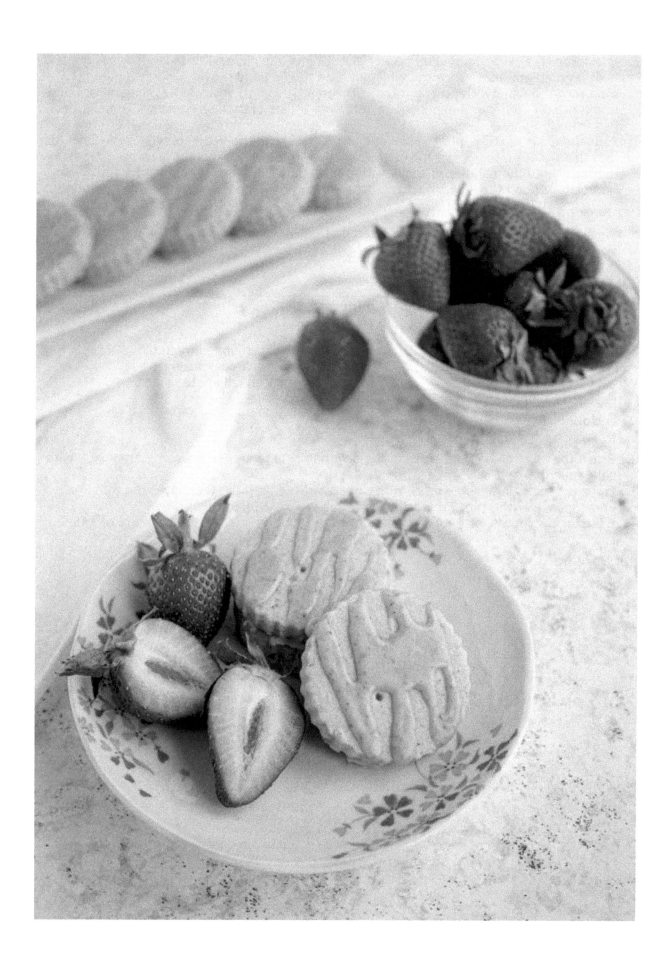

Chapter 8 Sweets and Desserts

Blackberry Lemon Panna Cotta

Prep time: 20 minutes | Cook time: 10 minutes | Serves 2

Ingredients:

¾ cup half-and-half, divided
1 teaspoon unflavored powdered gelatin
½ cup heavy cream
3 tablespoons sugar
1 teaspoon lemon zest

1 tablespoon freshly squeezed lemon juice
1 teaspoon lemon extract
½ cup fresh blackberries
Lemon peels to garnish (optional)

Directions:

1. Place ¼ cup of half-and-half in a small bowl.
2. Sprinkle the gelatin powder evenly over the half-and-half and set it aside for 10 minutes to hydrate.
3. In a saucepan, combine the remaining ½ cup of half-and-half, the heavy cream, sugar, lemon zest, lemon juice, and lemon extract. Heat the mixture over medium heat for 4 minutes, or until it's barely simmering—don't let it come to a full boil. Remove from the heat.
4. When the gelatin is hydrated (it will look like applesauce), add it into the warm cream mixture, whisking as the gelatin melts.
5. If there are any remaining clumps of gelatin, strain the liquid or remove the lumps with a spoon.
6. Pour the mixture into 2 dessert glasses or stemless wineglasses and refrigerate for at least 6 hours, or up to overnight.
7. Serve with the fresh berries and garnish with some strips of fresh lemon peel, if desired.

Per Serving

calories: 422 | fat: 33g | protein: 6g
carbs: 28g | fiber: 2g | sodium: 64mg

Strawberry Shortbread Cookies

Prep time: 20 minutes | Cook time: 10 minutes | Makes 3 dozen cookies

Ingredients:

2 cups cornstarch
1½ cups all-purpose flour
2 teaspoons baking powder
1 teaspoon baking soda
1 cup (2 sticks) cold butter, cut into 1-inch cubes
⅔ cup sugar

4 large egg yolks
2 tablespoons brandy
1 teaspoon vanilla extract
½ teaspoon salt
2 cups strawberry preserves
Confectioners' sugar, for sprinkling

Directions:

1. In a bowl, combine the cornstarch, flour, baking powder, and baking soda and mix together. Using your hands or 2 forks, mix the butter and sugar just until combined, with small pieces of butter remaining.
2. Add the egg yolks, brandy, vanilla, and salt, stirring slowly until all ingredients are blended together. If you have a stand mixer, you can mix these ingredients together with the paddle attachment and then finish mixing by hand, but it is not required.
3. Wrap the dough in plastic wrap and place in a resealable plastic bag for at least 1 hour.
4. Preheat the oven to 350ºF (180ºC).
5. Roll the dough to ¼-inch thickness and cut, placing 12 cookies on a sheet. Bake the sheets one at a time on the top rack of the oven for 12 to 14 minutes.
6. Let the cookies cool completely and top with about 1 tablespoon of strawberry preserves.
7. Sprinkle with confectioners' sugar.

Per Serving

calories: 157 | fat: 6g | protein: 1g
carbs: 26g | fiber: 0g | sodium: 132mg

Sesame Seed Cookies

Prep time: 10 minutes | Cook time: 15 minutes | Makes 14 to 16 cookies

Ingredients:

1 cup sesame seeds, hulled
1 cup sugar
8 tablespoons (1

stick) salted butter, softened
2 large eggs
1¼ cups flour

Directions:

1. Preheat the oven to 350ºF (180ºC). Toast the sesame seeds on a baking sheet for 3 minutes. Set aside and let cool.
2. Using a mixer, cream together the sugar and butter.
3. Add the eggs one at a time until well-blended.
4. Add the flour and toasted sesame seeds and mix until well-blended.
5. Drop spoonfuls of cookie dough onto a baking sheet and form them into round balls, about 1-inch in diameter, similar to a walnut.
6. Put in the oven and bake for 5 to 7 minutes or until golden brown.
7. Let the cookies cool and enjoy.

Per Serving

calories: 218 | fat: 12g | protein: 4g
carbs: 25g | fiber: 2g | sodium: 58mg

Buttery Almond Cookies

Prep time: 5 minutes | Cook time: 10 minutes | Serves 4 to 6

Ingredients:

½ cup sugar
8 tablespoons (1 stick) room temperature salted butter
1 large egg

1½ cups all-purpose flour
1 cup ground almonds or almond flour

Directions:

1. Preheat the oven to 375ºF (190ºC).
2. Using a mixer, cream together the sugar and butter.
3. Add the egg and mix until combined.
4. Alternately add the flour and ground almonds, ½ cup at a time, while the mixer is on slow.

5. Once everything is combined, line a baking sheet with parchment paper. Drop a tablespoon of dough on the baking sheet, keeping the cookies at least 2 inches apart.
6. Put the baking sheet in the oven and bake just until the cookies start to turn brown around the edges, about 5 to 7 minutes.

Per Serving

calories: 604 | fat: 36g | protein: 11g
carbs: 63g | fiber: 4g | sodium: 181mg

Cream Cheese and Ricotta Cheesecake

Prep time: 5 minutes | Cook time: 1 hour | Serves 8 to 10

Ingredients:

2 (8-ounce / 227-g) packages full-fat cream cheese
1 (16-ounce / 454-g) container full-fat ricotta cheese
1½ cups granulated

sugar
1 tablespoon lemon zest
5 large eggs
Nonstick cooking spray

Directions:

1. Preheat the oven to 350ºF (180ºC).
2. Using a mixer, blend together the cream cheese and ricotta cheese.
3. Blend in the sugar and lemon zest.
4. Blend in the eggs; drop in 1 egg at a time, blend for 10 seconds, and repeat.
5. Line a 9-inch springform pan with parchment paper and nonstick spray. Wrap the bottom of the pan with foil. Pour the cheesecake batter into the pan.
6. To make a water bath, get a baking or roasting pan larger than the cheesecake pan. Fill the roasting pan about ⅓ of the way up with warm water. Put the cheesecake pan into the water bath. Put the whole thing in the oven and let the cheesecake bake for 1 hour.
7. After baking is complete, remove the cheesecake pan from the water bath and remove the foil. Let the cheesecake cool for 1 hour on the countertop. Then put it in the fridge to cool for at least 3 hours before serving.

Per Serving

calories: 489 | fat: 31g | protein: 15g
carbs: 42g | fiber: 0g | sodium: 264mg

Honey Walnut Baklava

Prep time: 30 minutes | Cook time: 1 hour | Serves 6 to 8

Ingredients:

2 cups very finely chopped walnuts or pecans
1 teaspoon cinnamon
1 cup (2 sticks) unsalted butter,

melted
1 (16-ounce / 454-g) package phyllo dough, thawed
1 (12-ounce / 340-g) jar honey

Directions:

1. Preheat the oven to 350ºF (180ºC).
2. In a bowl, combine the chopped nuts and cinnamon.
3. Using a brush, butter the sides and bottom of a 9-by-13-inch inch baking dish.
4. Remove the phyllo dough from the package and cut it to the size of the baking dish using a sharp knife.
5. Place one sheet of phyllo dough on the bottom of the dish, brush with butter, and repeat until you have 8 layers.
6. Sprinkle ⅓ cup of the nut mixture over the phyllo layers. Top with a sheet of phyllo dough, butter that sheet, and repeat until you have 4 sheets of buttered phyllo dough.
7. Sprinkle ⅓ cup of the nut mixture for another layer of nuts. Repeat the layering of nuts and 4 sheets of buttered phyllo until all the nut mixture is gone. The last layer should be 8 buttered sheets of phyllo.
8. Before you bake, cut the baklava into desired shapes; traditionally this is diamonds, triangles, or squares.
9. Bake the baklava for 1 hour or until the top layer is golden brown.
10. While the baklava is baking, heat the honey in a pan just until it is warm and easy to pour.
11. Once the baklava is done baking, immediately pour the honey evenly over the baklava and let it absorb it, about 20 minutes. Serve warm or at room temperature.

Per Serving

calories: 1235 | fat: 89g | protein: 18g
carbs: 109g | fiber: 7g | sodium: 588mg

Pound Cake with Citrus Glaze

Prep time: 10 minutes | Cook time: 45 minutes | Serves 8

Ingredients:

Cake:

Nonstick cooking spray
1 cup sugar
⅓ cup extra-virgin olive oil
1 cup unsweetened almond milk

1 lemon, zested and juiced
2 cups all-purpose flour
1 teaspoon baking soda
1 teaspoon salt

Glaze:

1 cup powdered sugar
1 to 2 tablespoons freshly squeezed

lemon juice
½ teaspoon vanilla extract

Directions:

1. Preheat the oven to 350ºF (180ºC). Line a 9-inch loaf pan with parchment paper and coat the paper with nonstick cooking spray.
2. In a large bowl, whisk together the sugar and olive oil until creamy. Whisk in the milk and lemon juice and zest. Let it stand for 5 to 7 minutes.
3. In a medium bowl, combine the flour, baking soda, and salt. Fold the dry ingredients into the milk mixture and stir just until incorporated.
4. Pour the batter into the prepared pan and smooth the top. Bake until a toothpick or skewer inserted into the middle comes out clean with a few crumbs attached, about 45 minutes.
5. Remove the cake from the oven and cool for at least 10 minutes in the pan. Transfer to a cooling rack placed over a baking sheet and cool completely.
6. Make the Glaze
7. In a small bowl, whisk together the powdered sugar, lemon juice, and vanilla until smooth. Pour the glaze over the cooled cake, allowing the excess to drip off the cake onto the baking sheet beneath.

Per Serving

calories: 347 | fat: 9g | protein: 4g
carbs: 64g | fiber: 1g | sodium: 481mg

Creamy Rice Pudding

Prep time: 5 minutes | Cook time: 45 minutes | Serves 6

Ingredients:

1¼ cups long-grain rice

5 cups unsweetened almond milk

1 cup sugar

1 tablespoon rose water or orange blossom water

1 teaspoon cinnamon

Directions:

1. Rinse the rice under cold water for 30 seconds.
2. Put the rice, milk, and sugar in a large pot. Bring to a gentle boil while continually stirring.
3. Turn the heat down to low and let simmer for 40 to 45 minutes, stirring every 3 to 4 minutes so that the rice does not stick to the bottom of the pot.
4. Add the rose water at the end and simmer for 5 minutes.
5. Divide the pudding into 6 bowls. Sprinkle the top with cinnamon. Cool for at least 1 hour before serving. Store in the fridge.

Per Serving

calories: 323 | fat: 7g | protein: 9g
carbs: 56g | fiber: 1g | sodium: 102mg

Apple Pie Pockets

Prep time: 5 minutes | Cook time: 15 minutes | Serves 6

Ingredients:

1 organic puff pastry, rolled out, at room temperature

1 Gala apple, peeled and sliced

¼ cup brown sugar

⅛ teaspoon ground

cinnamon

⅛ teaspoon ground cardamom

Nonstick cooking spray

Honey, for topping

Directions:

1. Preheat the oven to 350ºF (180ºC).
2. Cut the pastry dough into 4 even discs. Peel and slice the apple. In a small bowl, toss the slices with brown sugar, cinnamon, and cardamom.
3. Spray a muffin tin very well with nonstick cooking spray. Be sure to spray only the muffin holders you plan to use.

4. Once sprayed, line the bottom of the muffin tin with the dough and place 1 or 2 broken apple slices on top. Fold the remaining dough over the apple and drizzle with honey.
5. Bake for 15 minutes or until brown and bubbly.

Per Serving

calories: 250 | fat: 15g | protein: 3g
carbs: 30g | fiber: 1g | sodium: 98mg

Baked Pears with Mascarpone Cheese

Prep time: 10 minutes | Cook time: 20 minutes | Serves 2

Ingredients:

2 ripe pears, peeled

1 tablespoon plus 2 teaspoons honey, divided

1 teaspoon vanilla, divided

¼ teaspoon ginger

¼ teaspoon ground coriander

¼ cup minced walnuts

¼ cup mascarpone cheese

Pinch salt

Directions:

1. Preheat the oven to 350ºF (180ºC) and set the rack to the middle position. Grease a small baking dish.
2. Cut the pears in half lengthwise. Using a spoon, scoop out the core from each piece. Place the pears with the cut side up in the baking dish.
3. Combine 1 tablespoon of honey, ½ teaspoon of vanilla, ginger, and coriander in a small bowl. Pour this mixture evenly over the pear halves.
4. Sprinkle walnuts over the pear halves.
5. Bake for 20 minutes, or until the pears are golden and you're able to pierce them easily with a knife.
6. While the pears are baking, mix the mascarpone cheese with the remaining 2 teaspoons honey, ½ teaspoon of vanilla, and a pinch of salt. Stir well to combine.
7. Divide the mascarpone among the warm pear halves and serve.

Per Serving

calories: 307 | fat: 16g | protein: 4g
carbs: 43g | fiber: 6g | sodium: 89mg

Fig Crostini with Mascarpone

Prep time: 10 minutes | Cook time: 10 minutes | Serves 6 to 8

Ingredients:

1 long French baguette
4 tablespoons (½ stick) salted butter, melted
1 (8-ounce / 227-

g) tub mascarpone cheese
1 (12-ounce / 340-g) jar fig jam or preserves

Directions:

1. Preheat the oven to 350ºF (180ºC).
2. Slice the bread into ¼-inch-thick slices.
3. Arrange the sliced bread on a baking sheet and brush each slice with the melted butter.
4. Put the baking sheet in the oven and toast the bread for 5 to 7 minutes, just until golden brown.
5. Let the bread cool slightly. Spread about a teaspoon or so of the mascarpone cheese on each piece of bread.
6. Top with a teaspoon or so of the jam. Serve immediately.

Per Serving

calories: 445 | fat: 24g | protein: 3g
carbs: 48g | fiber: 5g | sodium: 314mg

Orange Mug Cake

Prep time: 10 minutes | Cook time: 2 minutes | Serves 2

Ingredients:

6 tablespoons flour
2 tablespoons sugar
½ teaspoon baking powder
Pinch salt
1 teaspoon orange zest
1 egg
2 tablespoons olive oil

2 tablespoons freshly squeezed orange juice
2 tablespoons unsweetened almond milk
½ teaspoon orange extract
½ teaspoon vanilla extract

Directions:

1. In a small bowl, combine the flour, sugar, baking powder, salt, and orange zest.
2. In a separate bowl, whisk together the egg, olive oil, orange juice, milk, orange extract, and vanilla extract.

3. Pour the dry ingredients into the wet ingredients and stir to combine. The batter will be thick.
4. Divide the mixture into two small mugs that hold at least 6 ounces / 170 g each, or 1 (12-ounce / 340-g) mug.
5. Microwave each mug separately. The small ones should take about 60 seconds, and one large mug should take about 90 seconds, but microwaves can vary. The cake will be done when it pulls away from the sides of the mug.

Per Serving

calories: 302 | fat: 17g | protein: 6g
carbs: 33g | fiber: 1g | sodium: 117mg

Vanilla Cake Bites

Prep time: 10 minutes | Cook time: 45 minutes | Makes 24 bites

Ingredients:

1 (12-ounce / 340-g) box butter cake mix
½ cup (1 stick) butter, melted
3 large eggs, divided

1 cup sugar
1 (8-ounce / 227-g) cream cheese
1 teaspoon vanilla extract

Directions:

1. Preheat the oven to 350ºF (180ºC).
2. To make the first layer, in a medium bowl, blend the cake mix, butter, and 1 egg. Then, pour the mixture into the prepared pan.
3. In a separate bowl, to make layer 2, mix together sugar, cream cheese, the remaining 2 eggs, and vanilla and pour this gently over the first layer. Bake for 45 to 50 minutes and allow to cool.
4. Cut the cake into 24 small squares.

Per Serving

calories: 160 | fat: 8g | protein: 2g
carbs: 20g | fiber: 0g | sodium: 156mg

Cranberry Orange Loaf

Prep time: 20 minutes | Cook time: 45 minutes | Makes 1 loaf

Ingredients:

Dough:

3 cups all-purpose flour
1 (¼-ounce / 7-g) package quick-rise yeast
½ teaspoon salt
⅛ teaspoon ground cinnamon
⅛ teaspoon ground cardamom
½ cup water
½ cup almond milk
⅓ cup butter, cubed

Cranberry Filling:

1 (12-ounce / 340-g) can cranberry sauce
½ cup chopped walnuts
2 tablespoons grated orange zest
2 tablespoons orange juice

Directions:

1. In a large bowl, combine the flour, yeast, salt, cinnamon, and cardamom.
2. In a small pot, heat the water, almond milk, and butter over medium-high heat. Once it boils, reduce the heat to medium-low. Simmer for 10 to 15 minutes, until the liquid thickens.
3. Pour the liquid ingredients into the dry ingredients and, using a wooden spoon or spatula, mix the dough until it forms a ball in the bowl.
4. Put the dough in a greased bowl, cover tightly with a kitchen towel, and set aside for 1 hour.
5. To make the cranberry filling: In a medium bowl, mix the cranberry sauce with walnuts, orange zest, and orange juice in a large bowl.
6. Assemble the Bread
7. Roll out the dough to about a 1-inch-thick and 10-by-7-inch-wide rectangle.
8. Spread the cranberry filling evenly on the surface of the rolled-out dough, leaving a 1-inch border around the edges. Starting with the long side, tuck the dough under with your fingertips and roll up the dough tightly. Place the rolled-up dough in an "S" shape in a bread pan.
9. Allow the bread to rise again, about 30 to 40 minutes.
10. Preheat the oven to 350ºF (180ºC).
11. Bake in a preheated oven, 45 minutes.

Per Serving

calories: 704 | fat: 26g | protein: 12g
carbs: 111g | fiber: 6g | sodium: 448mg

Pomegranate Blueberry Granita

Prep time: 5 minutes | Cook time: 10 minutes | Serves 2

Ingredients:

1 cup frozen wild blueberries
1 cup pomegranate or pomegranate
blueberry juice
¼ cup sugar
¼ cup water

Directions:

1. Combine the frozen blueberries and pomegranate juice in a saucepan and bring to a boil. Reduce the heat and simmer for 5 minutes, or until the blueberries start to break down.
2. While the juice and berries are cooking, combine the sugar and water in a small microwave-safe bowl. Microwave for 60 seconds, or until it comes to a rolling boil. Stir to make sure all of the sugar is dissolved and set the syrup aside.
3. Combine the blueberry mixture and the sugar syrup in a blender and blend for 1 minute, or until the fruit is completely puréed.
4. Pour the mixture into an 8-by-8-inch baking pan or a similar-sized bowl. The liquid should come about ½ inch up the sides. Let the mixture cool for 30 minutes, and then put it into the freezer.
5. Every 30 minutes for the next 2 hours, scrape the granita with a fork to keep it from freezing solid.
6. Serve it after 2 hours, or store it in a covered container in the freezer.

Per Serving

calories: 214 | fat: 0g | protein: 1g
carbs: 54g | fiber: 2g | sodium: 15mg

Fruit and Nut Dark Chocolate Bark

Prep time: 15 minutes | Cook time: 5 minutes | Serves 2

Ingredients:

2 tablespoons chopped nuts (almonds, pecans, walnuts, hazelnuts, pistachios, or any combination of those)
3 ounces (85 g) good-quality dark

chocolate chips (about ⅔ cup)
¼ cup chopped dried fruit (apricots, blueberries, figs, prunes, or any combination of those)

Directions:

1. Line a sheet pan with parchment paper.
2. Place the nuts in a skillet over medium-high heat and toast them for 60 seconds, or just until they're fragrant.
3. Place the chocolate in a microwave-safe glass bowl or measuring cup and microwave on high for 1 minute. Stir the chocolate and allow any unmelted chips to warm and melt. If necessary, heat for another 20 to 30 seconds, but keep a close eye on it to make sure it doesn't burn.
4. Pour the chocolate onto the sheet pan. Sprinkle the dried fruit and nuts over the chocolate evenly and gently pat in so they stick.
5. Transfer the sheet pan to the refrigerator for at least 1 hour to let the chocolate harden.
6. When solid, break into pieces. Store any leftover chocolate in the refrigerator or freezer.

Per Serving

calories: 284 | fat: 16g | protein: 4g
carbs: 39g | fiber: 2g | sodium: 2mg

Grilled Fruit Skewers

Prep time: 15 minutes | Cook time: 10 minutes | Serves 2

Ingredients:

⅔ cup prepared labneh, or, if making your own, ⅔ cup full-fat plain Greek yogurt
2 tablespoons honey
1 teaspoon vanilla extract

Pinch salt
3 cups fresh fruit cut into 2-inch chunks (pineapple, cantaloupe, nectarines, strawberries, plums, or mango)

Directions:

1. If making your own labneh, place a colander over a bowl and line it with cheesecloth. Place the Greek yogurt in the cheesecloth and wrap it up. Put the bowl in the refrigerator and let sit for at least 12 to 24 hours, until it's thick like soft cheese.
2. Mix honey, vanilla, and salt into labneh. Stir well to combine and set it aside.
3. Heat the grill to medium (about 300ºF / 150ºC) and oil the grill grate. Alternatively, you can cook these on the stovetop in a heavy grill pan (cast iron works well).
4. Thread the fruit onto skewers and grill for 4 minutes on each side, or until fruit is softened and has grill marks on each side.
5. Serve the fruit with labneh to dip.

Per Serving

calories: 292 | fat: 6g | protein: 5g
carbs: 60g | fiber: 4g | sodium: 131mg

Chocolate Dessert Hummus

Prep time: 15 minutes | Cook time: 0 minutes | Serves 2

Ingredients:

Caramel:

2 tablespoons coconut oil
1 tablespoon maple syrup

1 tablespoon almond butter
Pinch salt

Hummus:

½ cup chickpeas, drained and rinsed
2 tablespoons unsweetened cocoa powder
1 tablespoon maple syrup, plus more to taste

2 tablespoons almond milk, or more as needed, to thin
Pinch salt
2 tablespoons pecans

Directions:

Make the Caramel

1. To make the caramel, put the coconut oil in a small microwave-safe bowl. If it's solid, microwave it for about 15 seconds to melt it.
2. Stir in the maple syrup, almond butter, and salt.
3. Place the caramel in the refrigerator for 5 to 10 minutes to thicken.

Make the Hummus

1. In a food processor, combine the chickpeas, cocoa powder, maple syrup, almond milk, and pinch of salt, and process until smooth. Scrape down the sides to make sure everything is incorporated.
2. If the hummus seems too thick, add another tablespoon of almond milk.
3. Add the pecans and pulse 6 times to roughly chop them.
4. Transfer the hummus to a serving bowl and when the caramel is thickened, swirl it into the hummus. Gently fold it in, but don't mix it in completely.
5. Serve with fresh fruit or pretzels.

Per Serving

calories: 321 | fat: 22g | protein: 7g | carbs: 30g | fiber: 6g | sodium: 100mg

Berry and Honey Compote

Prep time: 5 minutes | Cook time: 2 to 5 minutes | Serves 2 to 3

Ingredients:

½ cup honey
¼ cup fresh berries

2 tablespoons grated orange zest

Directions:

1. In a small saucepan, heat the honey, berries, and orange zest over medium-low heat for 2 to 5 minutes, until the sauce thickens, or heat for 15 seconds in the microwave. Serve the compote drizzled over pancakes, muffins, or French toast.

Per Serving

calories: 272 | fat: 0g | protein: 1g | carbs: 74g | fiber: 1g | sodium: 4mg

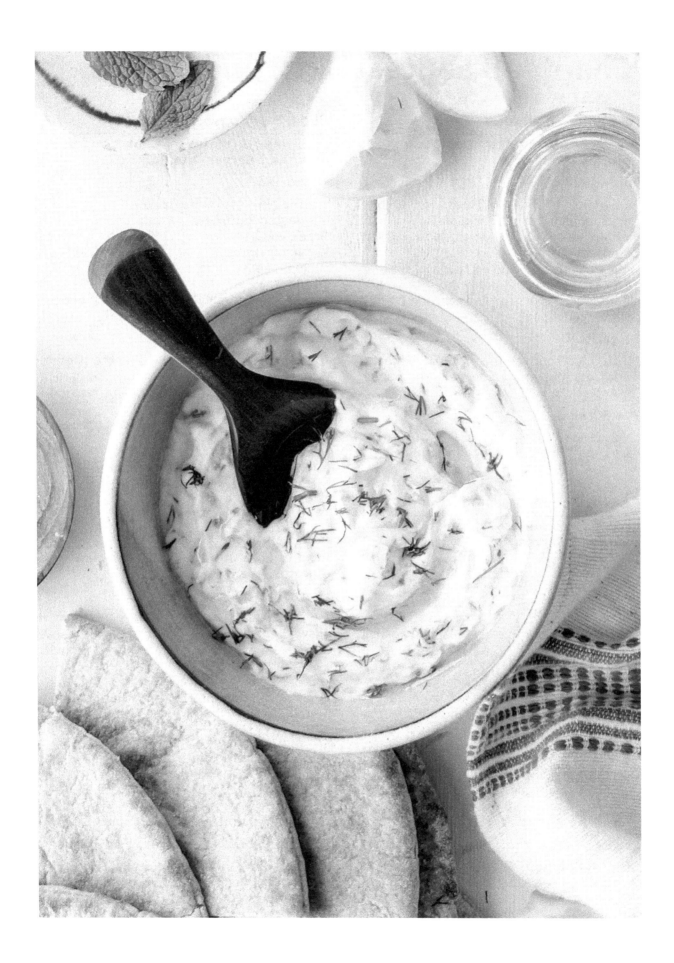

Chapter 9 Sauces, Dips, and Dressings

Red Wine Vinaigrette

Prep time: 5 minutes | Cook time: 0 minutes | Serves 2

Ingredients:

¼ cup plus 2 tablespoons extra-virgin olive oil
2 tablespoons red wine vinegar
1 tablespoon apple cider vinegar
2 teaspoons honey

2 teaspoons Dijon mustard
½ teaspoon minced garlic
⅛ teaspoon kosher salt
⅛ teaspoon freshly ground black pepper

Directions:

1. In a jar, combine the olive oil, vinegars, honey, mustard, garlic, salt, and pepper and shake well.

Per Serving

calories: 386 | fat: 41g | protein: 0g
carbs: 6g | fiber: 0g | sodium: 198mg

Creamy Yogurt Dressing

Prep time: 5 minutes | Cook time: 0 minutes | Serves 3

Ingredients:

1 cup plain, unsweetened, full-fat Greek yogurt
½ cup extra-virgin olive oil
1 tablespoon apple cider vinegar
½ lemon, juiced
1 tablespoon chopped fresh

oregano
½ teaspoon dried parsley
½ teaspoon kosher salt
¼ teaspoon garlic powder
¼ teaspoon freshly ground black pepper

Directions:

1. In a large bowl, combine the yogurt, olive oil, vinegar, lemon juice, oregano, parsley, salt, garlic powder, and pepper and whisk well.

Per Serving

calories: 402 | fat: 40g | protein: 8g
carbs: 4g | fiber: 0g | sodium: 417mg

Cucumber Yogurt Dip

Prep time: 5 minutes | Cook time: 0 minutes | Serves 2 to 3

Ingredients:

1 cup plain, unsweetened, full-fat Greek yogurt
½ cup cucumber, peeled, seeded, and diced
1 tablespoon freshly squeezed lemon

juice
1 tablespoon chopped fresh mint
1 small garlic clove, minced
Salt and freshly ground black pepper, to taste

Directions:

1. In a food processor, combine the yogurt, cucumber, lemon juice, mint, and garlic. Pulse several times to combine, leaving noticeable cucumber chunks.
2. Taste and season with salt and pepper.

Per Serving

calories: 128 | fat: 6g | protein: 11g
carbs: 7g | fiber: 0g | sodium: 47mg

Oregano Cucumber Dressing

Prep time: 5 minutes | Cook time: 0 minutes | Serves 2

Ingredients:

1½ cups plain, unsweetened, full-fat Greek yogurt
1 cucumber, seeded and peeled
½ lemon, juiced and zested

1 tablespoon dried, minced garlic
½ tablespoon dried dill
2 teaspoons dried oregano
Salt, to taste

Directions:

1. In a food processor, combine the yogurt, cucumber, lemon juice, garlic, dill, oregano, and a pinch of salt and process until smooth. Adjust the seasonings as needed and transfer to a serving bowl.

Per Serving

calories: 209 | fat: 10g | protein: 18g
carbs: 14g | fiber: 2g | sodium: 69mg

Orange Dijon Dressing

Prep time: 5 minutes | Cook time: 0 minutes | Serves 2

Ingredients:

¼ cup extra-virgin olive oil
2 tablespoons freshly squeezed orange juice
1 orange, zested
1 teaspoon garlic powder

¾ teaspoon za'atar seasoning
½ teaspoon salt
¼ teaspoon Dijon mustard
Freshly ground black pepper, to taste

Directions:

1. In a jar, combine the olive oil, orange juice and zest, garlic powder, za'atar, salt, and mustard. Season with pepper and shake vigorously until completely mixed.

Per Serving

calories: 283 | fat: 27g | protein: 1g
carbs: 11g | fiber:2 g | sodium: 597mg

Arugula Walnut Pesto

Prep time: 5 minutes | Cook time: 0 minutes | Serves 8 to 10

Ingredients:

6 cups packed arugula
1 cup chopped walnuts
½ cup shredded Parmesan cheese

2 garlic cloves, peeled
½ teaspoon salt
1 cup extra-virgin olive oil

Directions:

1. In a food processor, combine the arugula, walnuts, cheese, and garlic and process until very finely chopped. Add the salt. With the processor running, stream in the olive oil until well blended.
2. If the mixture seems too thick, add warm water, 1 tablespoon at a time, until smooth and creamy. Store in a sealed container in the refrigerator.

Per Serving (2 tablespoons)

calories: 296 | fat: 31g | protein: 4g
carbs: 2g | fiber: 1g | sodium: 206mg

Tarragon Grapefruit Dressing

Prep time: 5 minutes | Cook time: 0 minutes | Serves 4 to 6

Ingredients:

½ cup avocado oil mayonnaise
2 tablespoons Dijon mustard
1 teaspoon dried tarragon or 1 tablespoon chopped fresh tarragon

Zest and juice of ½ grapefruit (about 2 tablespoons juice)
½ teaspoon salt
¼ teaspoon freshly ground black pepper
1 to 2 tablespoons water (optional)

Directions:

1. In a large mason jar or glass measuring cup, combine the mayonnaise, Dijon, tarragon, grapefruit zest and juice, salt, and pepper and whisk well with a fork until smooth and creamy. If a thinner dressing is preferred, thin out with water.

Per Serving (2 tablespoons)

calories: 86 | fat: 7g | protein: 1g
carbs: 6g | fiber: 0g | sodium: 390mg

Tahini Dressing

Prep time: 5 minutes | Cook time: 0 minutes | Serves 8 to 10

Ingredients:

½ cup tahini
¼ cup freshly squeezed lemon juice (about 2 to 3 lemons)
¼ cup extra-virgin

olive oil
1 garlic clove, finely minced or ½ teaspoon garlic powder
2 teaspoons salt

Directions:

1. In a glass mason jar with a lid, combine the tahini, lemon juice, olive oil, garlic, and salt. Cover and shake well until combined and creamy. Store in the refrigerator for up to 2 weeks.

Per Serving (2 tablespoons)

calories: 121 | fat: 12g | protein: 2g
carbs: 2g | fiber: 1g | sodium: 479mg

Bagna Cauda

Prep time: 5 minutes | Cook time: 20 minutes | Serves 8 to 10

Ingredients:

½ cup extra-virgin olive oil
4 tablespoons (½ stick) butter
8 anchovy fillets, very finely chopped

4 large garlic cloves, finely minced
½ teaspoon salt
½ teaspoon freshly ground black pepper

Directions:

1. In a small saucepan, heat the olive oil and butter over medium-low heat until the butter is melted.
2. Add the anchovies and garlic and stir to combine. Add the salt and pepper and reduce the heat to low. Cook, stirring occasionally, until the anchovies are very soft and the mixture is very fragrant, about 20 minutes.
3. Serve warm, drizzled over steamed vegetables, as a dipping sauce for raw veggies or cooked artichokes, or use as a salad dressing. Store leftovers in an airtight container in the refrigerator for up to 2 weeks.

Per Serving (2 tablespoons)

calories: 181 | fat: 20g | protein: 1g | carbs: 1g | fiber: 0g | sodium: 333mg

Apple Cider Dressing

Prep time: 5 minutes | Cook time: 0 minutes | Serves 2

Ingredients:

2 tablespoons apple cider vinegar
$1/_3$ lemon, juiced
$1/_3$ lemon, zested

Salt and freshly ground black pepper, to taste

Directions:

1. In a jar, combine the vinegar, lemon juice, and zest. Season with salt and pepper, cover, and shake well.

Per Serving

calories: 4 | fat: 0g | protein: 0g | carbs: 1g | fiber: 0g | sodium: 0mg

Herbed Olive Oil

prep time: 5 minutes | Cook time: 0 minutes | Serves 2

Ingredients:

½ cup extra-virgin olive oil
1 teaspoon dried basil
1 teaspoon dried parsley

1 teaspoon fresh rosemary leaves
2 teaspoons dried oregano
⅛ teaspoon salt

Directions:

1. Pour the oil into a small bowl and stir in the basil, parsley, rosemary, oregano, and salt while whisking the oil with a fork.

Per Serving

calories: 486 | fat: 54g | protein:1 g | carbs: 2g | fiber: 1g | sodium: 78mg

Easy Tzatziki Sauce

Prep time: 5 minutes | Cook time: 0 minutes | Serves 2

Ingredients:

1 medium cucumber, peeled, seeded and diced
½ teaspoon salt, divided, plus more
½ cup plain, unsweetened, full-fat Greek yogurt

½ lemon, juiced
1 tablespoon chopped fresh parsley
½ teaspoon dried minced garlic
½ teaspoon dried dill
Freshly ground black pepper, to taste

Directions:

1. Put the cucumber in a colander. Sprinkle with ¼ teaspoon of salt and toss. Let the cucumber rest at room temperature in the colander for 30 minutes.
2. Rinse the cucumber in cool water and place in a single layer on several layers of paper towels to remove the excess liquid.
3. In a food processer, pulse the cucumber to chop finely and drain off any extra fluid.
4. Pour the cucumber into a mixing bowl and add the yogurt, lemon juice, parsley, garlic, dill, and the remaining ¼ teaspoon of salt. Season with salt and pepper to taste and whisk the ingredients together. Refrigerate in an airtight container.

Per Serving

calories: 77 | fat: 3g | protein: 6g | carbs: 6g | fiber: 1g | sodium: 607mg

Marinara Sauce

Prep time: 15 minutes | Cook time: 40 minutes | Makes 8 cups

Ingredients:

1 small onion, diced
1 small red bell pepper, stemmed, seeded and chopped
2 tablespoons plus ¼ cup extra-virgin olive oil, divided
2 tablespoons butter
4 to 6 garlic cloves, minced
2 teaspoon salt, divided

½ teaspoon freshly ground black pepper
2 (32-ounce / 907-g) cans crushed tomatoes (with basil, if possible), with their juices
½ cup thinly sliced basil leaves, divided
2 tablespoons chopped fresh rosemary
1 to 2 teaspoons crushed red pepper flakes (optional)

Directions:

1. In a food processor, combine the onion and bell pepper and blend until very finely minced.
2. In a large skillet, heat 2 tablespoons olive oil and the butter over medium heat. Add the minced onion, and red pepper and sauté until just starting to get tender, about 5 minutes.
3. Add the garlic, salt, and pepper and sauté until fragrant, another 1 to 2 minutes.
4. Reduce the heat to low and add the tomatoes and their juices, remaining ¼ cup olive oil, ¼ cup basil, rosemary, and red pepper flakes (if using). Stir to combine, then bring to a simmer and cover. Cook over low heat for 30 to 60 minutes to allow the flavors to blend.
5. Add remaining ¼ cup chopped fresh basil after removing from heat, stirring to combine.

Per Serving (1 cup)

calories: 256 | fat: 20g | protein: 4g | carbs: 19g | fiber: 5g | sodium: 803mg

Appendix 1: Measurement Conversion Chart

VOLUME EQUIVALENTS(DRY)

US STANDARD	METRIC (APPROXIMATE)
1/8 teaspoon	0.5 mL
1/4 teaspoon	1 mL
1/2 teaspoon	2 mL
3/4 teaspoon	4 mL
1 teaspoon	5 mL
1 tablespoon	15 mL
1/4 cup	59 mL
1/2 cup	118 mL
3/4 cup	177 mL
1 cup	235 mL
2 cups	475 mL
3 cups	700 mL
4 cups	1 L

VOLUME EQUIVALENTS(LIQUID)

US STANDARD	US STANDARD (OUNCES)	METRIC (APPROXIMATE)
2 tablespoons	1 fl.oz.	30 mL
1/4 cup	2 fl.oz.	60 mL
1/2 cup	4 fl.oz.	120 mL
1 cup	8 fl.oz.	240 mL
1 1/2 cup	12 fl.oz.	355 mL
2 cups or 1 pint	16 fl.oz.	475 mL
4 cups or 1 quart	32 fl.oz.	1 L
1 gallon	128 fl.oz.	4 L

TEMPERATURES EQUIVALENTS

FAHRENHEIT(F)	CELSIUS(C) (APPROXIMATE)
225 °F	107 °C
250 °F	120 °C
275 °F	135 °C
300 °F	150 °C
325 °F	160 °C
350 °F	180 °C
375 °F	190 °C
400 °F	205 °C
425 °F	220 °C
450 °F	235 °C
475 °F	245 °C
500 °F	260 °C

WEIGHT EQUIVALENTS

US STANDARD	METRIC (APPROXIMATE)
1 ounce	28 g
2 ounces	57 g
5 ounces	142 g
10 ounces	284 g
15 ounces	425 g
16 ounces (1 pound)	455 g
1.5 pounds	680 g
2 pounds	907 g

Appendix 2: Recipe Index

CPSIA information can be obtained
at www.ICGtesting.com
Printed in the USA
LVHW101410170321
681763LV00011B/403